English & Spanish Medical Words & Phrases

Fourth Edition

Pacific
WITHDRAWN
University

English & Spanish Medical Words & Phrases

Fourth Edition

Wolters Kluwer | Lippincott Williams & Wilkins
Health

Philadelphia · Baltimore · New York · London
Buenos Aires · Hong Kong · Sydney · Tokyo

STAFF

Publisher
Judith A. Schilling McCann, RN, MSN

Editorial Director
David Moreau

Clinical Director
Joan M. Robinson, RN, MSN

Art Director
Mary Ludwicki

Senior Managing Editor
Jaime Stockslager Buss, MSPH, ELS

Editorial Project Manager
Liz Schaeffer

Clinical Project Manager
Kate Stout, RN, MSN, CCRN

Editors
Maureen Haggerty, Ruth Steinhauer

Copy Editor
Karl Schaeffer

Designer
Linda Jovinelly Franklin

Digital Composition Services
Diane Paluba (manager),
Joyce Rossi Biletz (senior desktop
assistant), Donna S. Morris (senior
desktop assistant)

**Associate Manufacturing
Manager**
Beth J. Welsh

Editorial Assistants
Megan L. Aldinger, Karen J. Kirk,
Jeri O'Shea, Linda K. Ruhf

Indexer
Judith Young

ENG4010807

**Library of Congress
Cataloging-in-Publication Data**

English & Spanish medical words & phrases. — 4th ed.
    p. ; cm.
  Includes indexes.
  1. Medicine—Dictionaries. 2. Spanish language—Dictionaries—English. 3. Spanish language—Conversation and phrase books (for medical personnel) I. Title: English and Spanish medical words and phrases.
  [DNLM: 1. Medicine—Phrases—English. 2. Medicine—Phrases—Spanish. 3. Medicine—Terminology—English. 4. Medicine—Terminology—Spanish. W 15 E58 2008]
  R121.E575 2008
  610.3—dc22
ISBN-13: 978-1-58255-673-4 (alk. paper)
ISBN-10: 1-58255-673-3 (alk. paper)
                                        2007018691

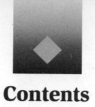

Contents

Appendices

Indexes

Translator and consultants

Spanish translator

Etcetera Language Group, Inc.
Washington, D.C.

Consultants

Diane M. Elmore, RN, MSN, FNP-C
Nursing Faculty, Family Nurse Practitioner
Great Basin College
Elko, Nev.

Lieutenant Commander Manual D. Leal, PA-C, MPAS
Senior Medical Officer
Branch Medical Clinic, Naval Training Center
San Diego, Calif.

Paul Mathews, RRT, PhD
Associate Professor, Respiratory Care, Physical Therapy
University of Kansas Medical Center
Kansas City

Gabriel Ortiz, MPAS, PA-C
Physician's Assistant
Allergy and Asthma Research Center of El Paso (Tex.)

Monica Narvaez Ramirez, RN, MSN
Nursing Instructor
University of the Incarnate Word School of Nursing and Health
Professions
San Antonio, Tex.

Richard R. Roach, MD, FACP
Assistant Professor of Internal Medicine
Michigan State University Kalamazoo Center for Medical Studies
Kalamazoo

Maria E. Rodriguez, RN, BS, CMSRN
Director of Education
Kindred Hospital
San Diego, Calif.

Christy M. Smith, APRN, MSN, BC
Affiliate Faculty
University of Phoenix (Ariz.)
Regis University
Denver, Colo.

Leigh Ann Trujillo, RN, BSN
Nurse Educator
St. James Hospital and Health Centers
Olympia Fields, Ill.

Patricia Van Tine, RN, MA, CPT
Nursing Faculty
Mt. San Jacinto College
Menifee, Calif.

Daniel T. Vetrosky, PhD, PA-C
Assistant Professor
University of South Alabama
Mobile

Trinidad Villaruel, RN, MSN
Clinical Nurse Specialist
Children's Hospital of New York
New York-Presbyterian-Columbia University

Contributors to previous editions

Glafyra Ennis, PhD

Marjorie S. Ramirez, RN,C, MA, EDM, CNA

Helen Gonzales-Kranzel, ARNP, MSN, MBA, CCRN

How to use this book

English & Spanish Medical Words & Phrases, Fourth Edition, is a portable, quick-reference resource with a handy format especially designed for use by English-speaking health care professionals with Spanish-speaking patients or by Spanish-speaking health care professionals with English-speaking patients. Featuring reliable translations for thousands of commonly used medical words and phrases, the book facilitates communication during every aspect of health care service.

Chapter 1 provides an overview of Spanish pronunciation and grammar, including nouns, pronouns, articles, possessives, contractions, prefixes and suffixes, comparisons, and spelling. It also provides a description of how to form masculine, feminine, and plural nouns, adjectives, and pronouns.

Subsequent chapters are arranged in a two-column format, with the English word or phrase in the left column and the Spanish equivalent in the right column.

Chapter 2 includes translations for commonly used terms and phrases, including greetings, general background information, days of the week, months and seasons of the year, holidays, numbers, units of time, colors, weights and measures, family members, anatomic terms, clothing, and hygiene supplies.

Chapter 3 contains patient-teaching terms and phrases, including admission, preoperative, and postoperative instructions; liability issues; tests and procedures; diabetic teaching; and drug administration.

Chapter 4 reviews common diagnostic tests, therapies, treatments, equipment, and drugs.

Chapter 5 lists frequently used medical equipment and supplies, such as assistive devices, I.V. therapy equipment, maternity care equipment, and respiratory equipment.

Chapter 6 covers words related to nutrition and diet therapies, such as your patients' food allergies, special diets, and dietary habits.

Arranged according to body systems, chapters 7 through 20 guide the reader through a carefully conducted assessment of the patient's health problems, medical history, family history, usual health patterns, and psychosocial considerations. Each of these chapters also provides pertinent information on developmental concerns affecting pediatric, adolescent, pregnant, and elderly patients.

Anatomic illustrations throughout feature English and Spanish titles and captions.

The informative appendices include therapeutic drug classifications; postoperative tubes, catheters, and equipment; medication teaching phrases; home care phrases; and a new list of phrases related to complementary and alternative therapies. Two indexes (one in English, one in Spanish) round out the text.

1

Pronunciation and grammar

This chapter provides a quick review of pronunciation for letters of the Spanish alphabet as well as some helpful tips on grammar and spelling.

Overview of Spanish pronunciation

A	Similar to the **A** in **fAther**
B	Similar to the **B** in **aBnormal**
C	Similar to the English **C**; it is hard when it precedes A, O, or U (as in **esCape**), soft when it precedes E or I (as in **paCe**)
CH	Similar to the **CH** in **CHild**
CU	Similar to the **QU** in **QUestion**
D	Similar to the **D** in **Day** when it is at the beginning of a word; similar to the **TH** in **wiTH** when it is in the middle of a word or at the end of a word
E	Similar to the **E** in **sEpsis**; the Spanish E does not end with the glide of the English **EY** in **thEY**
F	Similar to the **F** in **perForate**
G	Similar to the **G** in **Gout** when it precedes A, O, U, or a consonant; similar to the **H** in **Hospital** when it precedes E or I
H	Always silent
I	Similar to the **I** in **salIne**; similar to the **EE** in **sEE**
J	Similar to the **H** in **Hospital**
K	Similar to the **K** in **maKeup**
L	Similar to the **L** in **sLeep**
LL	Similar to the **LL** in **miLLion** and the **YE** in **YEllow**
M	Similar to the **M** in **atoMic**
N	Similar to the **N** in **learNing**; similar to the **M** in **coMma** when it precedes B, P, or V; silent when it precedes M
Ñ	Similar to the **NI** in **oNIon**
O	Similar to the **O** in **lOw**
P	Similar to the **P** in **sPit**
Q	Similar to the **K** in **Key**
R	Similar to the **R** in **haiRy**
RR	Always trilled; note that spelling a word with one **r** or two **r**'s changes the meaning of the word, as in **pero** (but) and **perro** (dog), **caro** (expensive) and **carro** (wagon, cart, car), and **para** (for) and **parra** (grapevine)

1

S   Similar to the **S** in **ba*S*ement**
T   Similar to the **T** in **s*T*ent**
U   Similar to the **U** in **fl*U***
V   Same as the Spanish B; similar to the **B** in **sa*B*le**
X   Similar to the **X** in **fle*X***; similar to the **S** in **me*SS*age** when
       it precedes a consonant
Y   Similar to the **Y** in **bo*Y*friend**; similar to **EE** in **s*EE*** when it
       is used to denote the word *and*
Z   Similar to the **C** in **Ci*t*y, pre*C*ede**

Vowels in Spanish are almost always pronounced in the same way. Spanish vowels are short and tense. They are neither drawn out nor glided. Spanish vowels are divided into two categories: strong vowels (a, e, and o) and weak vowels (i and u). A combination of a strong and a weak vowel or two weak vowels is pronounced as a single syllable, forming a diphthong (an unsegmented gliding sound in which the weak sounds [i, u] can hardly be heard), such as **lengua, nueve, and biopsia.** However, a written accent over the weak vowel breaks the diphthong into two separate syllables, such as **día** and **sangría.** In Spanish, the meaning of a word can change with the addition of a written accent, as in **seria** (serious) and **sería** (would be), **continuo** (continuous) and **continuó** (he continued), and **papa** (potato, especially in Latin America) and **papá** (dad or daddy).

Grammar and usage tips

Nouns

Nouns in Spanish are either masculine or feminine.
Most nouns ending in O or medical words ending in MA are masculine.
Most nouns ending in A are feminine.

Exceptions to this rule include:
Mano is always feminine.
Día, herbicida, insecticida, pesticida, raticida, espermaticida, and *vermicida* are always masculine.

Plurals

In general, a Spanish word is made plural by adding an S or ES to the end of the word.
Add an S when the word ends in an unaccented vowel.
Add an S when the word ends with an accented A, E, or O.
Add an ES when the word ends in a consonant, Y, or accented I or U.

Pronouns

Pronouns in Spanish are either masculine or feminine. The *you* pronoun has two forms: familiar and formal.
Singular forms
     I—yo
     You—tú (familiar)

You—usted (formal); abbreviated Ud. *or* Vd.
He—él
She—ella
Plural forms
We—nosotros (masculine)
We—nosotras (feminine)
You—vosotros (familiar, masculine)
You—vosotras (familiar, feminine)
You—ustedes (formal); abbreviated Uds. *or* Vds.
They—ellos (masculine)
They—ellas (feminine)

Articles and adjectives

The articles *the, a,* and *an* and the adjectives *this, that, these,* and *those* can be either masculine or feminine, depending on the gender of the noun they modify. *That* and *those* also have different forms to denote distance.
The
la (feminine, singular)
el (masculine, singular)
las (feminine, plural)
los (masculine, plural)
A, an
un (masculine)
una (feminine)
This
este (masculine)
esta (feminine)
That (near)
ese (masculine)
esa (feminine)
That (far)
aquel (masculine)
aquella (feminine)
These
estos (masculine)
estas (feminine)
Those (near)
esos (masculine)
esas (feminine)
Those (far)
aquellos (masculine)
aquellas (feminine)

Possessives

Like pronouns, the possessives used in Spanish are masculine or feminine and singular or plural. *Your* also has two forms: familiar and formal.
Singular forms
My—mi (singular)

My—mis (plural)
Your—tu (familiar)
Your—su (formal)
His—su
Her—su
Our—nuestro (masculine)
Our—nuestra (feminine)
Their—su

Plural forms

My—mis
Your—tus (familiar)
Your—sus (formal)
His—sus
Her—sus
Our—nuestros (masculine)
Our—nuestras (feminine)
Their—sus

Contractions

When the article *el* (the, masculine singular) is preceded by the preposition *a* (to, at) or *de* (of, from, about), you must form a contraction. For "to the," use *al*. For "of the," use *del*.

I am going to the doctor this afternoon—*Voy al doctor esta tarde.*

The people of the State of New York—*El pueblo del Estado de Nueva York*

Prefixes and suffixes

Special prefixes and suffixes may be added to Spanish words to denote certain things.

To denote the opposite meaning of the original word, add *des-* to the beginning of the word.

To denote the diminutive, such as slight or less, use *-ito, ita.*

To denote the augmentative, such as very, use *-ísimo, -ísima.*

To denote an adverb ending in -LY, add *-mente* to the feminine form of the adjective.

To denote a noun ending in -TY, such as in quantity or faculty, use *-dad* or *-tad.*

To denote the location where something is made or sold, add *-ería* to the end of the word.

To denote the person who makes or sells the object, add *-ero* or *-era* to the end of the word.

Comparisons

When comparing things, use *que*. When comparing quantities, use *de*.

Spelling

Note that four letters in the Spanish alphabet are not included in the English alphabet: ñ, ch, ll, rr. The last three double letters cannot be hyphenated.

Stress and written accent marks

For most Spanish words, **stress** can be predicted based on the written form of the word.

- If a word ends in a **vowel, n,** or **s,** stress normally falls on the next-to-last syllable:
  fu**ma** nece**si**ta ejer**ci**cio be**bi**das **u**san cer**ve**za
- If a word ends in a consonant other than **n** or **s,** stress normally falls on the last syllable:
  us**ted** doc**tor** do**lor** dificul**tad** intesti**nal** tra**gar**
- Any exception to these two rules will include a **written accent mark** on the stressed syllable:
  fácil ca**fé** evacua**ción** a**quí** anti**sép**tico
- Accents distinguish one-syllable words from other words that sound similar:
  él (he)   **el** (the)   **sí** (yes)   **si** (if)   **tú** (you, familiar form)   **tu** (your, familiar form)
- Interrogative and exclamatory words include a written accent on the stressed vowel:
  ¿qué? (what)   **¿quién?** (who)   **¿dónde?** (where)   **¿cuándo?** (when)   **¡cómo no!** (of course)

2

Commonly used terms and phrases

Greetings and introductions

Hello	¡Hola!
Good morning	Buenos días
Good afternoon	Buenas tardes
Good evening	Buenas noches
Come in, please.	Pase Ud. por favor.
My name is _____.	Me llamo_____.
Who is the patient?	¿Quién es el (la) paciente?
What is your name?	¿Cómo se llama Ud.?
It's nice to meet you.	Mucho gusto en conocerle.
How are you?	¿Cómo está Ud.?
I need you to sign this form.	Necesito que Ud. firme este formulario.
Please	Por favor
Thank you	Gracias
Yes	Sí
No	No
Maybe	Quizás *or* Tal vez
Sometimes	A veces
Never	Nunca
Always	Siempre
Date	Fecha
Signature	Firma
Good-bye	Hasta luego *or* Adiós

General information

How are you feeling?	¿Cómo se siente Ud?

What time is it?	**¿Qué hora es?**
What day is it?	**¿Qué día es hoy?**
What is the date?	**¿En qué fecha estamos?**
Where are you?	**¿Dónde está Ud.?**
How old are you?	**¿Cuántos años tiene Ud.?**
Did you come alone?	**¿Vino Ud. solo(a)?**
Who brought you here?	**¿Quién le trajo hasta aquí?**
Where were you born?	**¿Dónde nació Ud.?**
Where do you live?	**¿Dónde vive Ud.?**
What is your address?	**¿Cuál es su dirección?**
Do you live alone?	**¿Vive Ud. solo(a)?**

Who lives with you?
- Parents?
    Mother?
    Father?
- Spouse?
- Children?
    Son?
    Daughter?
    Grandchildren?
- Uncle?
- Aunt?
- Grandfather?
- Grandmother?
- Cousin?
- Friend?
- Other relative?

¿Quién vive con Ud.?
- ¿Sus padres?
    ¿Su madre?
    ¿Su padre?
- ¿Su esposo(a)?
- ¿Sus hijos?
    ¿Su hijo?
    ¿Su hija?
    ¿Sus nietos?
- ¿Su tío?
- ¿Su tía?
- ¿Su abuelo?
- ¿Su abuela?
- ¿Su primo(a)?
- ¿Su amigo(a)?
- ¿Otro pariente?

Are you:
- single?
- married?
- divorced?
- widowed?
- separated?

¿Es Ud.:
- soltero(a)?
- casado(a)?
- divorciado(a)?
- viudo(a)?
- (Esta Ud.) separado(a)?

Do you have any children?
- How many?

¿Tiene Ud. hijos?
- ¿Cuántos?

Did you go to school?
- How many grades did you complete?
- Did you go to college?

¿Asistió Ud. a la escuela?
- ¿Cuántos grados completó Ud.?
- ¿Hizo Ud. estudios universitarios?

What is your religion?
- Baptist?
- Buddhist?
- Catholic?

¿Cuál es su religión?
- ¿Bautista?
- ¿Budista?
- ¿Católica?

– Christian Scientist?	– ¿Científico(a) cristiano(a)?
– Congregationalist?	– ¿Congregacionalista?
– Episcopalian?	– ¿Episcopal? (Anglicano[a])
– Evangelist?	– ¿Evangelista?
– Hindu?	– ¿Hindú?
– Jehovah's Witness?	– ¿Testigo de Jehová?
– Jewish?	– ¿Judío(a)?
– Lutheran?	– ¿Luterano(a)?
– Methodist?	– ¿Metodista?
– Muslim?	– ¿Musulmán (musulmana)?
– Presbyterian?	– ¿Presbiteriano(a)?
– Protestant?	– ¿Protestante?

Do you work outside the home?   **¿Trabaja Ud. fuera de casa?**

– What type of work do you do?	– ¿Qué tipo de trabajo realiza?
Accountant?	¿Contador(a)?
Architect?	¿Arquitecto(a)?
Banker?	¿Banquero(a)?
Bus driver?	¿Conductor(a) de camiones/autobuses?
Businessperson?	¿Persona de negocios?
Computer operator?	¿Operador(a) de computadoras?
Designer?	¿Diseñador(a)?
Doctor?	¿Doctor(a)?
Engineer?	¿Ingeniero(a)?
Factory worker?	¿Obrero(a) en una fábrica?
Farmer?	¿Campesino(a)?
Lawyer?	¿Abogado(a)?
Mechanic?	¿Mecánico?
Salesperson?	¿Vendedor(a)? *or* ¿Dependiente?
Secretary?	¿Secretario(a)?
Student?	¿Estudiante?
Taxi driver?	¿Chofer de taxi?
Teacher?	¿Maestro(a)?
Truck driver?	¿Camionero(a)?
Waiter?	¿Mesero?
Waitress?	¿Mesera?

Where do you work?   **¿Dónde trabaja Ud.?**

Do you have any hobbies?   **¿Tiene Ud. pasatiempos favoritos?**

– Movies?	– ¿Cine?
– Music?	– ¿Música?
– Painting?	– ¿Arte?
– Photography?	– ¿Fotografía?
– Reading?	– ¿Leer?
– Sewing?	– ¿Cocinar?
– Sports?	– ¿Deportes?
Baseball?	¿Béisbol?
Basketball?	¿Baloncesto?

Football?	¿Fútbol americano?
Golf?	¿Golf?
Hockey?	¿Hockey?
Running?	¿Correr?
Soccer?	¿Fútbol?
Tennis?	¿Tenis?
– Theater?	– ¿Teatro?

Days of the week

Monday	lunes
Tuesday	martes
Wednesday	miércoles
Thursday	jueves
Friday	viernes
Saturday	sábado
Sunday	domingo

Months of the year

January	enero
February	febrero
March	marzo
April	abril
May	mayo
June	junio
July	julio
August	agosto
September	septiembre
October	octubre
November	noviembre
December	diciembre

Seasons of the year

Spring	La primavera
Summer	El verano
Fall	El otoño
Winter	El invierno

Holidays

New Year's Day	El día de Año Nuevo
Valentine's Day	Día de San Valentín *or* Día de los enamorados
Passover	Pascua de los hebreos
Ash Wednesday	Miércoles de ceniza
Good Friday	Viernes Santo
Easter	Pascua de Resurrección
Memorial Day	Día de conmemoración de los Caídos en batalla
Fourth of July	El cuatro de julio
Labor Day	El día del trabajo
Rosh Hashanah	Rosh Hashanah
Yom Kippur	Yom Kipur
Halloween	Víspera de Todos los Santos
Thanksgiving	Día de acción de gracias
Hanukkah	Hanukkah
Christmas	Día de Navidad
Anniversary	Aniversario
Birthday	Cumpleaños

Cardinal numbers

1	Uno
2	Dos
3	Tres
4	Cuatro
5	Cinco
6	Seis
7	Siete
8	Ocho
9	Nueve
10	Diez
11	Once
12	Doce

13	Trece
14	Catorce
15	Quince
16	(Diez y seis *or)* dieciséis
17	(Diez y siete *or)* diecisiete
18	(Diez y ocho *or)* dieciocho
19	(Diez y nueve *or)* diecinueve
20	Veinte
21	Veintiuno (*or* veinte y uno)
22	Veintidós (*or* veinte y dos)
23	Veintitrés (*or* veinte y tres)
24	Veinticuatro (*or* veinte y cuatro)
25	Veinticinco (*or* veinte y cinco)
30	Treinta
40	Cuarenta
50	Cincuenta
60	Sesenta
70	Setenta
80	Ochenta
90	Noventa
100	Cien
1,000	Mil
10,000	Diez mil
100,000	Cien mil
100,000,000	Cien millones

Ordinal numbers

First	Primero(a)
Second	Segundo(a)
Third	Tercero(a)
Fourth	Cuarto(a)
Fifth	Quinto(a)
Sixth	Sexto(a)

Seventh	Séptimo(a)
Eighth	Octavo(a)
Ninth	Noveno(a)
Tenth	Décimo, diez (*in dates*)
Eleventh	Décimo primero *or* undécimo, once (*in dates*)
Twelfth	Décimo segundo *or* duodécimo, doce (*in dates*)
Thirteenth	Décimo tercero, trece (*in dates*)

Time expressions

Second	Segundo
Minute	Minuto
Fifteen minutes	Quince minutos
Thirty minutes	Treinta minutos
Hour	Hora
In the morning	Por la mañana
At noon	Al medio día
In the afternoon	Por la tarde
In the evening	Por la noche
At midnight	A medianoche
What time is it?	¿Qué hora es?

Meals

Breakfast	El desayuno
Lunch	El almuerzo
Midafternoon snack	La merienda
Dinner	La cena
Bedtime snack	Bocadillo nocturno

Colors

Black	Negro
Blue	Azul

Brown	Café *or* marrón
Gray	Gris
Green	Verde
Orange	Anaranjado *or* color naranja
Pink	Rosado
Purple	Morado
Red	Rojo
White	Blanco
Yellow	Amarillo

Antonyms

Alive/Dead	Vivo/Muerto
Better/Worse	Mejor/Peor
Central/Peripheral	Central/Periférico
Dark/Light	Oscuro/Claro
Fat/Thin	Gordo/Delgado
Flat/Raised	Plano/En relieve
Healthy/Sick	Saludable/Enfermo
Heavy/Light	Pesado/Ligero
High/Low	Alto/Bajo
Hot/Cold	Caliente/Frío
Large/Small	Grande/Pequeño
Long (length)/Short (length)	Largo (longitud)/Corto (longitud)
Loud/Soft	Fuerte/Suave
Many/Few	Muchos/Pocos
Open/Closed	Abierto/Cerrado
Painful/Painless	Doloroso/Indoloro
Regular/Irregular	Regular/Irregular
Smooth/Rough	Liso/Áspero
Soft/Hard	Blando/Duro
Sweet/Sour	Dulce/Agrio
Symmetric/Asymmetric	Simétrico/Asimétrico
Tall (height)/Short (height)	Alto (estatura)/Bajo (estatura)

Thick/Thin	Grueso/Fino
Weak/Strong	Débil/Fuerte
Wet/Dry	Mojado/Seco

Weights and measures

Centimeter	Centímetro
Circumference	Circunferencia
Cubic centimeter	Centímetro cúbico
Deciliter	Decilitro
Depth	Profundidad
Foot	Pie
Gram	Gramo
Height	Altitud
Inch	Pulgada
Kilogram	Kilo
Length	Longitud
Liter	Litro
Meter	Metro
Microgram	Microgramo
Milligram	Miligramo
Milliliter	Mililitro
Millimeter	Milímetro
Tablespoon	Cucharada
Teaspoon	Cucharadita
Volume	Volumen
Weight	Peso
Width	Ancho
Yard	Yarda

Anatomic terms

Abdomen	Abdomen *or* vientre
Ankle	Tobillo
Arm	Brazo
Back	Espalda

Breast	Seno
Buttocks	Nalgas
Calf	Pantorrilla
Cheek	Mejilla
Chest	Pecho
Ear	Oreja
Elbow	Codo
Eye	Ojo
Face	Cara
Finger	Dedo de la mano
Fingernail	Uña
Foot	Pie
Groin	Ingle
Gums	Encías
Hair	Cabello *or* pelo
Hand	Mano
Head	Cabeza
Heel	Talón
Hip	Cadera
Jaw	Mandíbula *or* quijada
Knee	Rodilla
Leg	Pierna
Lip	Labio
Mouth	Boca
Neck	Cuello
Nose	Nariz
Rectum	Recto
Shin	Espinilla de la pierna
Shoulder	Hombro
Skin	Piel
Stomach	Estómago
Thigh	Muslo
Throat	Garganta
Toe	Dedo del pie

Tongue	Lengua
Tooth	Diente
Wrist	Muñeca

Clothing

Coat	Abrigo
Dress	Vestido
Gloves	Guantes
Hat	Sombrero
Pajamas	Piyamas *or* pijamas
Robe	Bata
Shirt	Camisa
Shoes	Zapatos
Skirt	Falda
Slippers	Pantuflas
Socks	Calcetines
Stockings	Medias
Trousers	Pantalones
Underwear	Ropa interior

Hygiene supplies

Basin	Lavabo *or* lavamanos
Blanket	Manta (frazada)
Brush	Cepillo
Comb	Peine
Deodorant	Desodorante
Lotion	Loción
Mouthwash	Enjuague para la boca
Pillow	Almohada
Pillowcase	Funda de almohada
Razor	Navaja de afeitar
Sanitary napkin	Toalla higiénica *or* toalla femenina
Shampoo	Champú

Shaving cream	Crema de afeitar
Sheet	Sábana
Soap	Jabón
Tampon	Tampón
Toothbrush	Cepillo de dientes
Toothpaste	Pasta de dientes
Towel	Toalla
Washcloth	Toallita de mano
Water	Agua

3

Patient teaching

Hospital admission procedures

As part of the admission process, I will need:

– a _____ sample.
– a wound culture.
– to check your _____.
– to draw some blood.
– to examine you.

– to insert an I.V. line.

– to listen to your:
    heart.
    lungs.
    stomach.
– to measure your vital signs.
– to take your:
    temperature.
    blood pressure.
    pulse.
    respirations.
– to measure your height and weight.

Como parte del proceso de ingreso, voy a necesitar lo siguiente:

– una muestra de _____.
– un cultivo de su herida.
– examinarle la _____.
– extraerle un poco de sangre.
– tengo que hacerle un reconocimiento.
– le voy a colocar una vía intravenosa.
– le voy a escuchar:
    el corazón.
    los pulmones.
    el estómago.
– para tomarle los signos vitales.
– para tomarle:
    la temperatura.
    la presión sanguínea.
    el pulso.
    la respiración.
– para medirle su estatura y su peso.

Teaching a patient about a disorder

Describing the disorder

Descripción de la enfermedad

The doctor has diagnosed you with _____.

You have a(n):
– aneurysm.
– blockage.
– blood clot.
– broken blood vessel.
– damaged or diseased area.

El doctor le ha hecho el diagnóstico de _____.

Ud. tiene un(a):
– aneurisma.
– obstrucción.
– coágulo de sangre.
– ruptura en un vaso sanguíneo.
– región dañada o enferma.

– growth or tumor.
– hemorrhage.
– infection.
– muscle spasm.
– narrowing.
– ulcer.

As a result, your _____ is (are):

– not working or functioning properly.
– not working as well as it should.
– not working at all.
– working too hard.

– not producing enough _____.
– producing too much _____.
– not receiving enough oxygen or blood.

Here is some information about _____ for you to read.

We do not know what causes this condition.

Describing the treatment

Treating your condition involves:
– changing your diet.
– exercising.
– having a special procedure called a(n) _____.

– gaining weight.
– losing weight.
– taking medication.
– managing pain.
– undergoing physical therapy.
– having surgery.
– wearing a brace or splint.

– formación anormal o tumor.
– hemorragia.
– infección.
– espasmo muscular.
– restricción.
– úlcera.

En consecuencia, el órgano _____ de su cuerpo o sistema:

– no funciona o no funciona debidamente.
– no funciona eficazmente.

– no funciona para nada.
– funciona con demasiada dificultad.

– no produce suficiente_____.
– produce demasiado(a)_____.
– no recibe la suficiente cantidad de oxígeno o sangre.

Aquí tiene Ud. información acerca de _____ para que la lea.

No se sabe qué provoca esta afección.

Descripción del tratamiento

El tratamiento de su afección supone:
– cambio de dieta.
– ejercicio.
– que se le haga(n) un(os) procedimiento(s) especial(es) que se llama(n) _____.

– subir de peso.
– bajar de peso.
– medicamentos.
– dominar el dolor.
– recibir fisioterapia.
– realizarse una cirugía.
– usar una abrazadera o férula.

Preoperative teaching

Preparation for surgery

Your doctor has recommended surgery to correct your _____ problem.

Preparación para la cirugía

Su doctor ha recomendado cirugía para corregir su problema de _____.

The surgeon will discuss the surgery with you and your family.

El cirujano les explicará el procedimiento a Ud. y a su familia.

You may have a blood transfusion during or after surgery.

Se le puede realizar una transfusión de sangre durante o después de la cirguía.

You will need to sign a consent form to give permission for the blood transfusion.

Ud. tendrá que firmar un formulario de consentimiento para la transfusión de sangre.

You will need anesthesia during your surgery.

Ud. necesitará anestesia durante la cirugía.

Anesthesia will:
– keep you asleep during surgery.

La anestesia hara que:
– esté dormido(a) durante la cirugía.

– keep you from feeling pain.

– no sienta dolor.

There are two kinds of anesthesia: local and general.

Hay dos tipos de anestesia: local y general.

Sometimes doctors use both kinds of anesthesia.

A veces los doctores usan una combinación de ambas.

Local anesthesia will keep you from feeling pain in part of your body.

La anestesia local evitará que sienta dolor en una parte del cuerpo.

During the surgery, you will be:
– awake.
– asleep.

Durante la cirugía, Ud. estará:
– despierto(a).
– dormido(a).

General anesthesia will numb your entire body, including your breathing muscles.

La anestesia general le adormecerá todo el cuerpo, incluso los músculos respiratorios.

A breathing tube attached to a respirator will help you breathe.

Se colocará un tubo respiratorio en el respirador para ayudarlo a respirar.

The anesthesiologist inserts the breathing tube into your throat after you are asleep; the tube will probably be removed before you wake up.

El anestesiólogo insertará el tubo respiratorio en su garganta después de que usted se haya quedado dormido(a); es probable que usted se despierte.

If the tube is still in your throat when you wake up, it is because the anesthesia has not worn off or because you still need help to breathe.

Si sigue teniendo el tubo en la garganta cuando se despierta, es porque aún no se ha disipado la anestesia o porque todavía necesita ayuda para respirar.

The night before surgery:
- You will have an I.V. access placed in your arm if you do not already have one.

- You must not eat or drink anything:
    after midnight.
    _____ hour(s) before the test.
- Your _____ will need to be:
    shaved.
    cleaned.
    prepped.
- You will need to drink this solution to empty and clean your bowels.

- You may have a catheter inserted into your bladder to drain urine while you are unable to use the bathroom or bedpan.

Preventing complications after surgery

Patients can develop pneumonia, blood clots, infections, or other complications after surgery.

Here are some things you can do to prevent these complications.

This is an incentive spirometer.

You will use it after surgery to help you take deep breaths.

To use the incentive spirometer:
- Put the mouthpiece into your mouth.
- Breathe in or suck air into your mouth.
- Keep this arrow between these two lines as you breathe.

En la víspera de la cirugía:
- Se le tendrá que poner un acceso intravenoso en el brazo si es que todavía no lo tiene colocado.

- No puede Ud. tomar ni beber nada:
    después de la medianoche.
    _____ hora(s) antes del análisis.
- Se tendrá que:
    razurar.
    limpiar.
    preparar.
- Ud. tendrá que tomarse esta solución para vaciar y limpiar su intestino.

- Es posible que se le inserte un catéter en la vejiga para drenar orina mientras usted no pueda ir al baño o evacuar en una chala.

Cómo evitar complicaciones después de la cirugía

Los pacientes pueden sufrir neumonía, coágulos de sangre, infecciones, u otras complicaciones después de la cirugía.

Éstas son algunas de las maneras de evitar estas complicaciones.

Esto es un espirómetro de estímulo.

Ud. usará este aparato después de la cirugía para ayudarle a respirar profundamente.

Para usar el espirómetro de estímulo:
- Métase la boquilla en la boca.

- Aspire o ingrese aire en la boca.

- Mantenga esta flecha entre las dos rayas al aspirar.

– Try to move this arrow up to (number preset by respiratory therapist).

In addition to medications, there are other ways to relieve pain.

Splinting can help reduce pain caused by moving or coughing.

This is how to splint:
– Hold a pillow or large blanket firmly against your incision.

– Hug or squeeze the pillow or blanket tightly and push it into your incision as you move or cough.

Focus on things such as reading, meditating, watching television, or other activities to keep your mind off your pain.

Ask for pain medication about 30 minutes before major activities.

If the pain prevents you from moving, breathing, or coughing, ask for more pain medication.

You should be comfortable.

After surgery, it will be very important for you to:
– move.
– walk.
– sit up.
– take frequent deep breaths.

– cough.

Take about 10 deep breaths every hour.

– Trate de mover la flecha hasta el (número programado por el [la] terapeuta respiratorio[a]).

Además del medicamento, hay otros modos de aliviar el dolor.

El entablillador puede disminuir el dolor producido al moverse o al toser.

Así se entablilla:
– Coja una almohada o una manta grande y sujétela fuertemente contra la incisión.
– Apriétela o sosténgala fuertemente y empújela contra la incisión al moverse o al toser.

Concéntrese en pasatiempos como leer, meditar, mirar la televisión, u otras actividades para poder distraerse y no pensar en el dolor.

Pida Ud. un medicamento contra el dolor aproximadamente media hora antes de cualquier actividad fuerte.

Si el dolor no le permite moverse, respirar o toser, pida que se le dé más medicamento para el dolor.

Ud. debe estar cómodo(a).

Después de la cirugía es importante que Ud.:
– se mueva.
– camine.
– se incorpore/se siente.
– respire profundamente con frecuencia.
– tosa.

Respire a fondo diez veces por hora.

The morning of the surgery

You will receive a special pre-operative medication by injection or through your I.V. line.

You will need to urinate before we give you the preoperative medication.

The preoperative medication will:
– relax you.
– make you feel drowsy.

– give you a dry mouth.
– make your vision a little blurry.
– make you feel a little light-headed.

We will not give you all of your usual medications.

You will take only your _____ medication with a sip of water.

We will give you fluids through your I.V. line.

You may drink clear liquids or sips of water.

En la mañana de la cirugía

A Ud. se le dará un medicamento especial prequirúrgico por medio de una inyección o por via intravenosa (I.V.).

Ud. tendrá que orinar antes de que se le dé el medicamento prequirúrgico.

El medicamento prequirúrgico:

– lo (a) hará relajarse.
– lo (a) hará sentirse soñoliento(a).
– hará que sienta la boca seca.
– tenga la vista borrosa.
– hará sentirse un poco mareado(a) o confundido(a).

No le daremos sus medicamentos habituales.

Únicamente tomará Ud. su medicamento _____ con un sorbo de agua.

Se le darán líquidos por vía intravenosa (I.V.).

Ud. puede tomar líquidos claros o sorbos de agua.

Postoperative teaching

After surgery

You will wake up in the post-anesthesia care unit (PACU).

You will stay in the PACU for about an hour or until your vital signs are stable, you are awake, and you are breathing on your own.

You may receive oxygen through a:
– nasal cannula.

Después de la cirugía

Ud. despertará en la sala de post-anestesia (PACU, por su sigla en inglés).

Ud. permanecerá en la sala de PACU durante alrededor una hora o hasta que sus signos vitales estén estables, estê despierfo y respire por sus propios medios.

Puede recibir oxígeno a través de una:
– cánula nasal.

– mask over your nose and mouth.

– máscara sobre la nariz y la boca.

You may have a tube, catheter, or other equipment. (See the appendix Postoperative tubes, catheters, and equipment.)

Ud. puede tener un tubo, un catéter, u otro aparato. (Vé el apéndice Tubos, catéteres, y equipos postquirúrgicos.)

When you wake up, you may feel:
– pain.
– nausea.
– dryness in your mouth.
– soreness in your throat.
– groggy.
– sleepy.
– uncomfortable.

Cuando Ud. despierte, puede sentir:
– dolor.
– náuseas.
– la boca seca.
– dolor de garganta.
– mareos.
– somnolencia.
– incomodidad.

Ask the nurse to give you medication for:
– nausea.
– pain.

Pídale a la enfermera que le dé medicamentos para:
– las náuseas.
– el dolor.

The nurse will closely monitor your vital signs.

La enfermera observará cuidadosamente sus signos vitales.

If the doctor wants to monitor you more closely, you may be transferred to the intensive care unit.

Si el doctor quiere observar sus signos vitales más detalladamente, Ud. irá a la unidad de terapia intensiva.

Medication teaching phrases

Introductory statements

Informe preliminar

I would like to give you:
– an injection.
– an I.V. medication.

– a liquid medication.
– a medicated cream or powder.

– a medication through your epidural catheter.
– a medication through your rectum.
– a medication through your _____ tube.
– a medication under your tongue.
– your pill(s).
– a suppository.

Quisiera darle un(a):
– inyección.
– medicamento por vía intravenosa.
– medicamento en forma líquida.
– medicamento en pomada o polvo.
– medicamento por el catéter epidural.
– medicamento por el recto.

– medicamento por su tubo_____.

– medicamento debajo de la lengua/sublingual.
– de sus píldoras.
– supositorio.

This is how you take this medication.

Así se toma este medicamento.

If you cannot swallow this pill, I can crush it and mix it in some:
– applesauce.
– pudding.
– yogurt.
– liquid.

Si Ud. no se puede tragar esta píldora, puedo aplastarla y mezclarla en:
– puré de manzana.
– pudín.
– yogur.
– un líquido.

If you cannot swallow this pill, I can get it in another form.

Si Ud. no se puede tragar esta píldora, puede obtenerla en otra forma.

If you cannot swallow this pill, you can crush it and mix it in soft food.

Si Ud. no se puede tragar la píldora, la puede moler y mezclar en un alimento blando.

I need to mix this medication in juice or water.

Tengo que mezclar este medicamento en jugo (zumo) o agua.

I need to give you this injection in your:
– abdomen.
– buttocks.
– hip.
– outer arm.
– thigh.

Tengo que ponerle esta inyección:
– en el abdomen.
– en las nalgas.
– en la cadera.
– en la parte superior del brazo.
– en el muslo.

I need to give you this medication through your I.V. line.

Tengo que darle este medicamento por vía intravenosa (I.V.).

Place this under your tongue.

Póngaselo debajo de la lengua.

You should feel some burning when this is under your tongue.

Ud. debería sentir ardor cuando se lo pone debajo de la lengua.

The burning indicates that the medication is working.

El ardor indica que el medicamento está haciendo efecto.

Some medications are coated with a special substance so they will not upset your stomach.

Algunos medicamentos están cubiertos con una sustancia especial para no provocarle trastornos estomacales.

Do not chew:
– enteric-coated pills.

– long-acting pills.
– capsules.
– medication you take under the tongue.

No masque:
– píldoras con recubrimiento entérico.
– píldoras de efecto prolongado.
– cápsulas.
– medicamentos sublinguales/que se colocan debajo de la lengua.

Ask your doctor or pharmacist whether you may:
– mix your medication with food or fluids.
– take your medication with food.

You must take your medication:
– after meals.
– before meals.
– on an empty stomach.
– with meals or food.

Skipping doses

If you skip or miss a dose:
– Take your medication as soon as you remember it.
– Do not take your medication until it is time for the next dose.
– Call the doctor if you are not sure whether you should take your medication.
– Do not take an extra dose.

Side effects

Some common side effects of _____ are:
– constipation
– diarrhea
– difficulty sleeping
– dry mouth
– fatigue
– headache
– itching
– light-headedness
– nausea
– poor appetite
– rash
– upset stomach
– weight loss or gain
– frequent urination.

These side effects:
– will go away after your body gets used to the medication.

– may continue as long as you take the medication.

Pregúntele a su doctor o farmacéutico si debería:
– mezclar su medicamento con un alimento o con líquidos.
– tomar su medicamento con alimento.

Debe tomar el medicamento:
– después de las comidas.
– antes de las comidas.
– con el estómago vacío.
– con las comidas o con un alimento.

Si se saltea (omite) una dosis

Si Ud. omite o se saltea una dosis:
– Tómela apenas se acuerde.

– Espere hasta la siguiente dosis.

– Llame al doctor si Ud. no está seguro(a) de si debe tomar el medicamento.
– No tome una dosis extra.

Efectos secundarios

Algunos efectos secundarios comunes de _____ son:
– estreñimiento
– diarrea
– dificultad para dormir
– boca seca
– fatiga
– dolor de cabeza
– comezón (picazón)
– mareo
– náuseas
– poco apetito
– erupción
– trastorno estomacal
– perdida o aumento de peso
– orinación frecuente.

Estos efectos secundarios:
– desaparecerán una vez que su cuerpo se acostumbre al medicamento.
– pueden continuar mientras Ud. tome el medicamento.

If these side effects bother you, speak to your doctor about changing your medication.

If you experience side effects of your medication, call your doctor right away.

Other concerns

Tell your doctor if you are pregnant or breast-feeding.

While you are taking this medication, ask your doctor if:

- you can safely take other over-the-counter medications.
- you can drink alcoholic beverages.
- your medications interact with each other.

Storing medication

You should keep your medication:
- in a cool, dry place.
- in the refrigerator.

Do not keep your medication:
- in a warm place or near heat.

- in the sun.
- in your pocket.
- in the bathroom medicine cabinet.

Si le molestan, hable con su doctor sobre un posible cambio de medicamento.

Si su medicamento le provoca efectos secundarios, llame a su doctor inmediatamente.

Otras preocupaciones

Dígale a su doctor si Ud. está embarazada o si amamanta.

Mientras Ud. tome este medicamento, pregúntele a su doctor si:

- puede tomar otros medicamentos de venta libre.
- puede tomar bebidas alcohólicas.
- sus medicamentos interactúan uno con el otro.

Cómo guardar los medicamentos

Ud. debería guardar sus medicamentos:
- en un lugar fresco y seco.
- en el refrigerador.

No guarde su medicamento:
- en un lugar cálido ni cerca de la calefacción.
- en el sol.
- en su bolsillo.
- en el botiquín del baño.

Diabetic teaching

Insulin preparation and administration

The doctor has ordered insulin for you.

To draw up insulin, follow these steps:
- Wipe the rubber top of the insulin bottle with alcohol.

- Remove the needle cap.

Cómo preparar y administrar la insulina

El doctor ha recetado insulina para Ud.

Para extraer la insulina, siga los siguientes pasos:
- Limpie la tapa de hule (goma) de la botella de insulina con alcohol.
- Quítele el capuchón a la aguja.

– Pull out the plunger until the end of the plunger in the barrel lines up with the number of units of insulin you need.

– Push the needle through the rubber top of the insulin bottle.

– Inject the air into the bottle.

– Without removing the needle, turn the bottle upside down.
– Withdraw the plunger until the end of the plunger lines up with the number of units of insulin you need.
– Gently pull the needle out of the bottle.

To mix insulin, follow these steps:
– Wipe the rubber tops of the insulin bottles with alcohol.

– Gently roll the bottle of cloudy insulin between your palms.

– Remove the needle cap.
– Pull out the plunger until the end of the plunger in the barrel lines up with the number of units of NPH or Lente insulin you need.
– Push the needle through the rubber top of the cloudy insulin bottle.
– Inject the air into the bottle.

– Remove the needle.
– Pull out the plunger until the end of the plunger in the barrel lines up with the number of units of clear regular insulin you need.
– Push the needle through the rubber top of the clear insulin bottle.
– Inject the air into the bottle.

– Without removing the needle, turn the bottle upside down.

– Saque el émbolo hasta que el otro extremo del émbolo en la cuba esté al nivel del número de unidades de insulina que Ud. necesita.
– Perfore con la aguja la tapa de hule (goma) de la botella de insulina.
– Inyecte el aire dentro de la botella.
– Sin sacar la aguja de la botella, póngala boca abajo.
– Retire el émbolo hasta que la insulina llegue al número de unidades que Ud. necesita.

– Retire la aguja de la botella suavemente.

Para mezclar la insulina siga los siguientes pasos:
– Limpie la tapa de hule (goma) de las botellas de insulina con alcohol.
– Suavemente mueva la botella de insulina turbia entre las palmas de las manos.
– Retire el capuchón de la aguja.
– Saque el émbolo hasta que el otro extremo del émbolo en el barril llegue a la cantidad de unidades de NPH o insulina Lente que Ud. necesita.
– Empuje la aguja por la tapa de goma (hule) de la botella de insulina turbia.
– Inyecte el aire dentro de la botella.
– Saque la aguja.
– Retire el émbolo hasta que el otro extremo del émbolo en el barril se alinee con la cantidad de unidades de insulina clara regular que Ud. necesita.
– Perfore con la aguja la tapa de goma de la botella de insulina clara.
– Inyecte el aire dentro de la botella.
– Sin sacar la aguja, coloque la botella boca abajo.

– Withdraw the plunger until it lines up with the number of units of clear regular insulin you need.

– Gently pull the needle out of the bottle.

– Push the needle into the cloudy (NPH or Lente) insulin without injecting anything into the bottle.

– Withdraw the plunger until you reach your total dosage of insulin in units (regular combined with NPH or Lente).

– We will practice this again.

– Retire el émbolo hasta que llegue a la cantidad de insulina regular clara que Ud. necesita.

– Suavemente saque la aguja de la botella.

– Inserte la aguja en la insulina (NPH o insulina Lente) sin inyectarla dentro de la botella.

– Retire el émbolo hasta que llegue a su dosis total de insulina en unidades (regular y NPH/Lente combinadas).

– Practicaremos esto juntos(as) otra vez.

Using a blood glucose monitor

El uso del monitor de glucosa en la sangre

The doctor wants you to measure your blood sugar level at home.

El doctor quiere que Ud. mida en casa su nivel de azúcar en sangre.

You will do this using a special machine called a blood glucose monitor.

Ud. realizará está operación por medio de un aparato especial que se llama monitor de glucosa en sangre.

To operate the blood glucose monitor, follow these steps:

Para operar el monitor de glucosa en sangre, siga estos pasos:

– Turn the machine on.

– Wash your hands with soap and water.

– Prick your finger with the lancet.

– Place a drop of blood onto the designated area on the strip.

– Put the strip into the monitor.

– The machine will count for _____ seconds.

– You can read your blood sugar number here.

– If the number is high:
    call your doctor.
    follow his or her directions.

– If the number is low:
    drink some orange juice.
    eat a carbohydrate such as candy.

    call your doctor.

– Encienda el aparato.

– Lávese las manos con agua y jabón.

– Pínchese el dedo con la lanceta.

– Ponga una gota de sangre en el área indicada de la tira.

– Coloque la tira en el monitor.

– El aparato contará por _____ segundos.

– Aquí puede leer su número de glucosa en sangre.

– Si indica un número alto:
    llame a su doctor.
    siga sus instrucciones.

– Si el número es bajo:
    tome jugo (zumo) de naranja.
    coma alimentos con carbohidratos, como las golosinas.
    llame a su doctor.

Symptoms of hypoglycemia and hyperglycemia	**Síntomas de hipoglucemia e hiperglucemia**

Signs and symptoms of low blood sugar are:
– shakiness
– nervousness
– hunger
– nausea
– light-headedness
– confusion.

Los síntomas de un nivel bajo de azúcar en sangre:
– temblores
– nerviosismo
– hambre
– náuseas
– mareos
– desorientación.

If you have signs or symptoms of low blood sugar:
– Check your blood sugar level.

– Drink some orange juice.
– Call your doctor. He or she may want to adjust the amount of medication you take.

Si Ud. tiene síntomas de un nivel bajo de azúcar en sangre:
– Controle su nivel de azúcar en sangre.
– Beba jugo (zumo) de naranja.
– Llame a su doctor. Es posible que él/ella quiera modificar la cantidad de medicamento que toma.

Signs and symptoms of high blood sugar are:
– thirst
– sleepiness
– frequent urination
– fruity smell to breath.

Síntomas de un nivel elevado de azúcar en sangre:
– sed
– somnolencia
– orinación frecuente
– olor a fruta en el aliento.

If you have signs or symptoms of high blood sugar:
– Check your blood sugar level.

– Call your doctor.

Si Ud. tiene síntomas de un alto nivel de azúcar en sangre:
– Controle su nivel de azúcar en sangre.
– Llame a su doctor.

Other discharge teaching

Teaching a patient to do a procedure	**Cómo instruir al paciente para que realice un procedimiento**

Your doctor wants you to learn how to:
– catheterize yourself.
– change your dressing.
– check your blood pressure.
– check your pulse.
– clean and replace your ostomy pouch.
– clean your wound.

Su doctor quiere que Ud. sepa como:
– introducirse un catéter.
– cambiar su vendaje.
– medir su presión sanguínea.
– tomarse el pulso.
– limpiar y cambiar su saco de ostomía.
– limpiarse la herida.

– draw up and mix your insulin.
– flush your:
    catheter.
    tube.
– give yourself an injection.
– monitor your blood sugar level.

– suction yourself through your tracheostomy.
Let me show you how to do it.

Let's practice together.

I want you to do it yourself.

Let me know if you have trouble:
– handling the equipment.
– seeing the directions.
– understanding the directions.

– sacar y mezclar su insulina.
– lavar con agua su:
    catéter.
    tubo.
– inyectarse.
– controlar su nivel de azúcar en sangre.
– succionar por sus medios a través de su traqueotomia.
Permítame enseñarle cómo hacerlo.

Vamos a ensayar junto(a)s.

Quiero que Ud. lo haga solo(a).

Dígame si Ud. tiene dificultad para:
– manejar el aparato.
– ver las instrucciones.
– comprender las instrucciones.

Teaching a patient to give a subcutaneous injection

Cómo enseñarle al (a la) paciente a apicarse una inyección subcutanea

To give yourself an injection, follow these steps:
– Draw up the medication.
– Replace the cap carefully.

– Pick an injection site. Be sure to change the site regularly.

– Clean the skin area with alcohol.
– Gently pinch up a little skin over the area.
– Stab the needle into your skin like a dart.
– Gently pull back on the plunger to see if there is any blood in the syringe.
– Using the plunger, steadily push the medication into your skin.

– Pull the needle out.
– Apply gentle pressure with the alcohol wipe.
– Throw away the needle in an appropriate receptacle.

Para aplicarse una inyección, siga estos pasos:
– Saque el medicamento.
– Coloque de nuevo la tapa con cuidado.
– Elija un lungar de inyección. Asegúrese de cambiar el lugar frecuentemente.
– Limpie el área de la piel con alcohol.
– Suavemente pellizque un poco de piel sobre el área.
– Inserte la aguja en su piel como si fuera un dardo.
– Con cuidado retire el émbolo para ver si hay sangre en la jeringa.
– Inserte firmemente con el émbolo el medicamento dentro de su piel.
– Saque la aguja.
– Ejerza presión suavemente con una toallita con alcohol.
– Deseche la aguja en un recipiente apropiado.

4

Common diagnostic tests, therapies, and treatments

General therapies and treatments

Instructions	Instrucciones
Bend backward.	Inclínese hacia atrás.
Bend forward.	Inclínese hacia adelante.
Do not talk.	No hable.
Lean backward.	Recuéstese.
Lean forward.	Inclínese hacia adelante.
Lie down.	Acuéstese.
Lie on your back.	Acuéstese boca arriba.
Lie on your: – left side. – right side.	Acuéstese sobre: – el lado izquierdo. – el lado derecho.
Lie on your stomach.	Acuéstese boca abajo.
Roll over.	Dese vuelta.
Say AAHH.	Diga AAAA.
Sit down.	Siéntese.
Sit up.	Enderécese.
Stand up.	Póngase de pie.
Turn to the side.	Voltéese hacia un lado.
Whisper.	Susurre.

Examinations	Reconocimientos

I'm going to examine your:
– skin.
– hair.
– nails.
– head and neck.
    head.
    nose.
    mouth.
	Le voy a examinar:
	– la piel.
	– el cabello.
	– las uñas.
	– la cabeza y el cuello.
	    la cabeza.
	    la nariz.
	    la boca.

throat.	la garganta.
neck.	el cuello.
eyes.	los ojos.
ears.	las orejas.
– respiratory system.	– el sistema respiratorio.
chest.	el pecho.
lungs.	los pulmones.
– cardiovascular system.	– el sistema cardiovascular.
heart.	el corazón.
pulse.	el pulso.
– gastrointestinal system.	– el sistema gastrointestinal.
abdomen.	el abdomen.
rectum.	el recto.
– urinary system.	– el sistema urinario.
bladder.	la vejiga.
kidneys.	los riñones.
– reproductive system.	– el sistema reproductor.
breasts.	las mamas *or* los senos .
pelvis.	la pelvis.
penis.	el pene.
testicles.	los testículos.
– nervous system.	– el sistema nervioso.
reflexes.	los reflejos.
– musculoskeletal system.	– el sistema músculo-esquelético.
back.	la espalda
arms.	los brazos.
legs.	las piernas.
– immune system.	– el sistema inmunológico.
– endocrine system.	– el sistema endocrino.

I am going to take your vital signs. / **Voy a tomarle los signos vitales.**

– Blood pressure — – La presión sanguínea
– Oxygen saturation — – La saturción de oxigeno
– Pulse — – El pulso
– Respirations — – La respiración
– Temperature — – La temperatura

I am going to take a blood sample. / **Voy a tomarle una muestra de sangre.**

You need to give me a urine specimen. / **Tiene que darme un espécimen de orina.**

I am going to inspect your _____. / **Le voy a inspeccionar_____.**

I'm going to listen to your _____. / **Le voy a auscultar_____.**

I'm going to push on your _____. / **Le voy a palpar_____.**

I'm going to tap on your _____.	Le voy a percutir_____.
Are you comfortable?	¿Está cómodo?
Does this hurt?	¿Le duele esto?
– Where does it hurt?	– ¿Dónde le duele?

Equipment

Measuring tape	Cinta para medir
Ophthalmoscope	Oftalmoscopio
Otoscope	Otoscopio
Penlight	Linterna de bolsillo
Pulse oximeter	Oxímetro del pulso
Scale	Báscula (balanza)
Sphygmomanometer	Esfigmomanómetro
Stethoscope	Estetoscopio
Syringe	Jeringa
Thermometer	Termómetro
Tongue blade	Depresor de lengua
Tuning fork	Diapasón
Vaginal speculum	Espéculo para la vagina
Visual acuity chart	Gráfica de la acuidad visual

Diagnostic tests

General laboratory tests

Análisis de laboratorio en general

Biopsy	Biopsia
Blood test	Análisis de la sangre
Blood culture	Cultivo sanguíneo
Computed tomography (CT)	Tomografía computarizada (TC)
Endoscopy	Endoscopia
Magnetic resonance imaging (MRI)	Formación de imágenes por resonancia magnética (MRI)
Ultrasound	Ecografia
X-ray	Radiografías

Head and neck	**La cabeza y el cuello**
Neck X-ray	Radiografías del cuello
Nose culture	Cultivo de la nariz
Skull X-ray	Radiografías del cráneo
Throat culture	Cultivo de la garganta

Eyes	**Los ojos**
Glaucoma test	Examen de glaucoma
Vision test	Examen de la vista

Ears	**Las orejas**
Hearing test	Examen de la audición

Respiratory system	**El sistema respiratorio**
Arterial blood gases	Gases de la sangre arterial
Bronchoscopy	Broncoscopia
Chest X-ray	Radiografías del tórax
Computed tomography (CT) scan of the chest	Tomografía computarizada (TC) del tórax
Lung scan	Visualización del pulmón por ecos de ultrasonidos
Pulmonary function tests	Reconocimiento de la función pulmonar
Pulse oximetry	Oximetría del pulso
Sputum culture	Cultivo de esputo

Cardiovascular system	**El sistema cardiovascular**
Arteriogram	Arteriograma
Blood test for:	Análisis de la sangre para:
– Cardiac enzymes	– Encimas cardiacas
– Cholesterol	– Colesterol
– Partial thromboplastin time	– Tiempo de tromblastina parcial
– Prothrombin time	– Tiempo de protrombina
– Triglycerides	– Triglicéridos
– Troponin	– Troponina
Cardiac catheterization	Cateterismo cardiaco
Cardiac monitoring	Monitoreo cardiaco
Echocardiogram	Ecocardiograma

Electrocardiogram	Electrocardiograma
Holter monitor	Monitor Holter
Stress test	Examen de estrés
Venogram	Venograma

Gastrointestinal system / Sistema gastrointestinal

Abdominal ultrasound	Ultrasonido abdominal
Barium enema	Enema de bario
Barium swallow	Papilla de bario
Blood test for: – Amylase – Liver enzymes	Análisis de la sangre para: – Amilasa – Enzimas hepáticas
Cholangiogram	Colangiograma
Cholecystogram	Colecistograma
Colonoscopy	Colonoscopia
Computed tomography (CT) scan of the abdomen	Tomografía computarizada (TC) ecografia del abdomen
Endoscopy	Endoscopía
Gastric analysis	Análisis gástrico
Gastroscopy	Gastroscopia
Liver biopsy	Biopsia del hígado
Sigmoidoscopy	Sigmoidoscopia
Spleen scan	Visualización del bazo por ecos de ultrasonidos
Stool culture	Cultivo de materia fecal
Upper GI series	Serie gastrointestinal superior

Urologic system / Sistema urológico

Blood test for: – Blood urea nitrogen (BUN) – Creatinine – Electrolytes	Análisis de la sangre para: – Nitrógeno y urea sanguínea – Creatinina – Electrolitos
Cystoscopy	Cistoscopia
Excretory urography	Urografía del sistema excretor
Renal biopsy	Cultivo renal
Retrograde pyelogram	Pielograma retrógrado
24-hour urine test	Análisis de orina de 24 horas
Urinalysis	Urinálisis

Urine culture	Cultivo de orina

Reproductive system

Sistema reproductivo

Breast biopsy	Biopsia de la mama
Breast examination	Examen mamario
Cervical biopsy	Biopsia cervical
Mammogram	Mamograma
Papanicolaou (Pap) test	Examen de Papanicolau
Pelvic examination	Reconocimiento pélvico
Pelvic ultrasound	Ecografía pélvica
Pregnancy test	Análisis de embarazo
Prostate examination	Examen de próstata
Prostatic biopsy	Biopsia de la próstata
Rectal examination	Reconocimiento del recto
Semen analysis	Análisis del semen
Vaginal culture	Cultivo vaginal

Neurologic system

El sistema neurológico

Brain scan	Visualización del cerebro por ecos de ultrasonidos
Cerebral arteriogram	Arteriograma cerebral
Computed tomography (CT) scan of the brain	Tomografía computarizada (TC) visualización del cerebro
Electroencephalogram (EEG)	Electroencefalograma
Lumbar puncture	Punción lumbar
Magnetic resonance imaging (MRI) of the brain	Imagen de resonancia magnética (IRM) del cerebro
Myelogram	Mielograma

Musculoskeletal system

El sistema músculo-esquelético

Arthroscopy	Artroscopia
Bone biopsy	Biopsia del hueso
Electromyogram	Electromiograma
Muscle biopsy	Biopsia del músculo
X-ray of:	Radiografías de:
– Ankle	– El tobillo
– Arm	– El brazo

– Back
– Elbow
– Foot
– Hand
– Hip
– Knee
– Leg
– Ribs
– Shoulder
– Wrist

– La espalda
– El codo
– El pie
– La mano
– La cadera
– La rodilla
– La pierna
– Las costillas
– El hombro
– La muñeca

Immune system and blood

El sistema inmunológico y la sangre

Allergy tests

Análisis de alergia

Blood test for:
– Blood cell count
   Differential blood cell count

   Red blood cell count

   White blood cell count

– Clotting time
– Hematocrit
– Hemoglobin
– Hepatitis B
– Human immunodeficiency virus (HIV)
– Platelet count

Análisis de la sangre para:
– Recuento sanguíneo
   Recuento diferencial de las células sanguíneas

   Recuento de los glóbulos rojos de la sangre

   Recuento de los glóbulos blancos de la sangre

– El tiempo de coagulación
– Hematocrito
– El nivel de hemoglobina
– Hepatitis tipo B
– Virus de inmunodeficiencia humana (VIH)
– Recuento de plaquetas

Bone marrow biopsy

Biopsia de la médula ósea

Endocrine system

Sistema endocrino

Analysis of:
– Adrenal function
– Ovarian function
– Parathyroid function
– Pancreatic function
– Pituitary function
– Testicular function
– Thyroid function

Análisis de:
– La función adrenal
– La función ovárica
– La función paratiroidea
– La función pancreática
– La función de la pituitaria
– La función testicular
– La función de la tiroides

Blood test for:
– Serum calcium level
– Serum glucose level
   Fasting glucose level

   Glucose tolerance
   Glycosylated hemoglobin level

Análisis sanguíneo para:
– Suero del nivel de calcio
– Suero del nivel de glucosa
   El nivel de glucosa en ayunas

   Tolerancia de glucosa
   El nivel de hemoglobina glucosilada

2-hour postprandial glucose level	El nivel de glucosa 2-horas posprandial
– Serum hormone levels	– Niveles del suero de hormonas
– Serum phosphorus concentration	– Concentración de suero de fósforo

Specialists

Anesthesiologist	Anestesista
Cardiologist	Cardiólogo
Dentist	Dentista
Dermatologist	Dermatólogo
Endocrinologist	Endocrinólogo
Gastroenterologist	Gastroenterólogo
Gynecologist	Ginecólogo
Hematologist	Hematólogo
Infectious disease specialist	Especialista en edefermedades infecciosas
Internist	Internista
Nephrologist	Nefrólogo
Neurologist	Neurólogo
Nutritionist	Nutricionista
Obstetrician	Obstetra
Oncologist	Oncólogo
Ophthalmologist	Oftalmólogo
Orthopedist	Ortopedista
Otolaryngologist	Otorrinonaringólogo
Pediatrician	Pedriatra
Psychiatrist	Psiquiatra
Psychologist	Psicólogo
Pulmonologist	Pulmonólogo
Radiologist	Radiólogo
Surgeon	Cirujano

Drug therapy

Routes	Vías
Inhalation	Inhalatoria
Intradermal	Intradérmica
Intramuscular	Intramuscular
Intravenous	Intravenosa
Oral	Oral
Rectal	Rectal
Subcutaneous	Subcutánea
Sublingual	Sublingual
Topical	Tópica
Transdermal	Transdérmica
Vaginal	Vaginal

Preparations	Preparaciones
Capsule	Cápsula
Cream	Pomada
Drops	Gotas
Elixir	Elixir
Enema	Enema
Infusion	Infusión
Injection	Inyección
Inhaler	Inhalador
Lotion	Loción
Lozenge	Pastilla
Ointment	Ungüento
Patch	Parche
Powder	Polvo
Spray	Atomizador
Suppository	Supositorio
Suspension	Suspensión
Syrup	Jarabe
Tablet	Tableta

Frequency

Once daily

Twice daily

Three times daily

Four times daily

In the morning

With meals

Before meals

After meals

Before bedtime

When you have_____

Only when you need it

Every four hours

Every six hours

Every eight hours

Every twelve hours

Storage

At room temperature

In the refrigerator

Out of direct sunlight

In a dry place

Away from heat

Away from children

Frecuencia

Una vez al día

Dos veces al día

Tres veces al día

Cuatro veces al día

Por la mañana

Con las comidas

Antes de las comidas

Después de las comidas

Antes de acostarse

Cuando Ud. tome_____

Sólo cuando lo necesite

Cada cuatro horas

Cada seis horas

Cada ocho horas

Cada doce horas

Almacenamiento

A temperatura ambiente

En el refrigerador

Fuera de la luz del sol directa

En un lugar seco

Lejos de la calefacción

Lejos del alcance de los niños

5

Medical equipment and supplies

Assistive devices

Cane

You will need to walk with a cane.
- Hold the cane on the unaffected side of your body.
- Hold the cane close to your body so you will not lean.
- Move the cane and the leg at the same time.

Bastón

Ud. necesitará andar con bastón.
- Sostenga el bastón del lado del cuerpo no afectado.
- Sostenga el bastón cerca del cuerpo para evitar inclinarse.
- Mueva el bastón y la pierna al mismo tiempo.

Walker

You will need to use a walker.

- Hold the handgrips firmly and equally.
- Advance the walker 6 to 8 inches.
- Step forward with the affected leg, then follow with the unaffected leg.
- Use your arms to support yourself.
- Make sure all your steps are the same length.

Andador

Ud. necesitará usar un andador.
- Sostenga las manijas firmemente y de modo parejo.
- Adelante el andador de seis a ocho pulgadas.
- Dé un paso con la pierna afectada primero y después con la pierna no afectada.
- Utilice los brazos para sostenerse.
- Asegúrese de que todos sus pasos tengan la misma extensión.

Cardiac care equipment

Electrocardiogram

You need to have an electrocardiogram so we can check your heart's electrical activity.

This is a cardiac monitor; it will help us monitor your

Electrocardiograma

Ud. necesita un electrocardiograma para que podamos observar la actividad eléctrica del corazón.

Éste es un monitor cardiaco, que nos ayudará a controlar

heartbeat and heart rhythm.	sus pulsaciones y su ritmo cardiaco.
You will be attached to the cardiac monitor while you are in this unit.	Ud. estará conectado al monitor cardiaco mientras esté en esta unidad.
I need to place these electrodes on your body.	Tengo que colocarle estos electrodos en el cuerpo.
Do not be frightened if you hear the alarms; they sometimes sound when you move.	No se asuste si oye las alarmas que a veces suenan cuando se mueve.

Pacemaker

Marcapasos

You have an abnormal heart rhythm.	Ud. tiene un ritmo cardiaco anormal.
You need a pacemaker.	Ud. necesita un marcapasos.
I am going to apply this external pacemaker.	Voy a ponerle este marcapasos externo.
I need to place a patch on your chest and back.	Necesito ponerle un parche en el tórax (pecho) y en la espalda.

I.V. therapy equipment

I.V. catheter and pump

I.V. catéter y bomba

I need to insert an I.V. into your arm.	Tengo que insertarle una intravenosa (I.V.) en el brazo.
This is an I.V. pump.	Ésta es una bomba I.V.
The I.V. pump will help control the way the medicine flows through your I.V.	La bomba I.V. ayudará a regular el flujo de medicamento por su intravenosa.
I am going to insert the I.V. catheter.	Voy a introducirle el catéter de I.V.
I need to apply a tourniquet around your arm. It will feel tight.	Tengo que ponerle un torniquete alrededor del brazo. Lo sentirá ajustado.
You're going to feel a needle stick.	Ud. va a sentir un piquete de aguja.
I need to place a bandage over the I.V. site.	Tengo que ponerle un vendaje en el lugar de la I.V.
Call me if you have pain, redness, or swelling at your I.V. site.	Llámeme si tiene dolor, enrojecimiento o hinchazón en el lugar de la I.V.

I.V. drug administration

You need to have an I.V. catheter inserted so medicine can flow into your body.

I need to flush your I.V. catheter to keep it open.

Administración de medicamentos por I.V.

Ud. necesita que se le ponga un catéter de I.V. para que los medicamentos ingresen a su cuerpo.

Tengo que enjuagar su catéter de I.V. para mantenerlo abierto.

Invasive devices

Arterial line

I need to insert an arterial line into your wrist to check your blood pressure.

I will give you a local anesthetic so you will not feel any pain when I insert the catheter.

I am going to take a sample of blood from your arterial line.

Línea arterial

Necesito insertarle una línea arterial en la muñeca para controlar la presión sanguínea.

Le daré una anestesia local antes de insertarle el catéter para que no sienta dolor en el momento de la inserción.

Voy a tomar una muestra de sangre de su línea arterial.

Central venous catheter

You need a central venous catheter so fluids can flow into your body.

We will give you a local anesthetic so you will not feel any pain when we insert the catheter.

I need to place a dressing over the site.

Catéter venoso central

Ud. necesita un catéter venoso central para que los fluidos puedan ingresar a su cuerpo.

Le daremos anestesia local antes de insertarle el catéter para que no sienta dolor en el momento de la inserción.

Necesito colocar una gasa sobre el lugar.

Pulmonary artery catheter

You need a catheter placed through a major vein into your heart.

This catheter will help us monitor how well your heart is pumping.

I am going to take readings from your catheter.

Catéter de la arteria pulmonar

Ud. necesita que se le ponga un catéter por una de las venas principales del corazón.

Este catéter arterial pulmonar nos ayudará a revisar el estado del bombeo cardiaco.

Voy a leer lo que marca su catéter.

Maternity care equipment

External fetal monitor

This is an external fetal monitor.

I will place this monitor around your abdomen.

This monitor will record your contractions and your baby's heartbeat.

Monitor fetal externo

Éste es un monitor fetal externo.

Lo pondré alrededor de su abdomen.

El monitor registrará sus contracciones y las pulsaciones de su bebé.

Fetoscope

This is a fetoscope.

I will place the fetoscope on your abdomen so I can listen to your baby's heartbeat.

Your baby's heartbeat is _____.

Fetoscopio

Éste es un fetoscopio.

Se lo pondré en el abdomen para escuchar los latidos de su criatura.

Las pulsaciones de su bebé son _____.

Internal fetal monitor

This is an internal fetal monitor.

A small instrument, called a probe, will be placed onto the baby's scalp.

The probe will not hurt you or your baby.

It will monitor your contractions and your baby's heartbeat.

Monitor fetal interno

Éste es un monitor fetal interno.

Se colocará un pequeño instrumento, llamado sonda en el cuero cabelludo de la criatura.

La sonda no dañará a su bebé.

Observará sus contracciones y las pulsaciones de su bebé.

Isolette

This is an isolette.

I will place your baby in the isolette to keep him warm.

Incubadora

Ésta es una incubadora.

Pondré a su criatura en la incubadora para mantenerlo abrigado.

Light therapy

Your baby is jaundiced.

Your baby will need to be placed under special lights to make his skin less yellow.

Terapia lumínica

Su criatura tiene ictericia.

Su bebé deberá estar bajo luces especiales que harán que su piel se vea menos amarillenta.

We will place patches over your baby's eyes to protect them.	Colocaremos parches en los ojos del bebé para protegerios.

Personal care equipment

Bedpan

Here is a bedpan. Use it if you need to move your bowels or urinate.

Do you need to use the bedpan?

Let me help you get on the bedpan.

Call me when you are finished with the bedpan.

Cuña

Aquí tiene una cuña por si Ud. tiene que evacuar.

¿Necesita usar la cuña?

Permitame ayudario a colocarse la cuña.

Llámeme cuando acabe de usar la cuña.

Bedside commode

Your doctor does not want you to walk to the bathroom.

I can get you a bedside commode.

Call me when you are finished using the commode. I will help you get back into bed.

Silla retrete al lado de la cama

Su doctor no quiere que camine hasta el baño.

Le puedo traer una silla retrete.

Llámeme cuando haya acabado de usar la silla retrete. Lo ayudaré a regresar a la cama.

Blanket

Do you need a blanket?

Cobija

¿Necesita una manta (cobija)?

Emesis basin

This is an emesis basin.

You can use this basin if you need to throw up.

Call me when you're finished using the basin.

Cubeta para vómitos

Aquí está una cubeta para vómito.

Ud. puede usar esta cubeta si tiene que vomitar.

Llámeme cuando haya acabado de usar la cubeta.

Enema

This is an enema.

You need an enema to help you move your bowels.
– Lie on your left side.

Enema

Éste es un enema.

Ud. necesita un enema para ayudarle a evacuar.
– Acuéstese del lado izquierdo.

– I'm going to put this tube into your rectum.

– Take a deep breath.

– Let me know if you feel cramping.

– Try to retain the fluid for five minutes.

– Let me know when you are ready to move your bowels.

– Voy a insertarle este tubo en el recto.

– Respire profundamente.

– Dígame por favor si siente retortijones.

– Trate Ud. de retener el líquido durante cinco minutos.

– Aviseme cuando esté listo para evacuar.

Urinal

This is a urinal.

Do you need to use the urinal?

Call me when you are finished using the urinal.

Orinal

Aquí está un orinal.

¿Necesita usar el orinal?

Llámeme cuando acabe de usar el orinal.

Respiratory care equipment

Chest tube

You need to have a tube inserted into your chest to reexpand your lung.

You need to have a tube inserted into your chest to drain fluid.

This tube will help your breathing.

We will give you a local anesthetic before we insert the tube.

Tubo para el pecho

Tengo que insertarle un tubo en el tórax para volver a expandir el pulmón.

Tengo que insertarle un tubo en el tórax para extraer líquido.

Este tubo le ayudará a respirar.

Le daremos anestesia local antes que le insertemos el tubo.

Croup tent

Your child needs to be placed in a croup tent.

The tent will provide warm mist and oxygen to help your child breathe.

Carpa de Croup

Es necesario poner a su hijo(a) en una cámara de Croup.

Le proveerá vapor tibio y oxígeno a su hijo(a) para ayudarle a respirar.

Incentive spirometer

This is an incentive spirometer.

It will help you take deep breaths.

Espirómetro de estímulo

Éste es un estímulo de espirometría.

Le ayudará a respirar profundamente.

Breathe in deeply, hold your breath, then breathe out.

Inhale profundamente, contenga la respiración, luego exhale.

You should use the incentive spirometer every hour while you are awake.

Ud. deberá usar el estímulo de espirometría cada hora mientras esté despierto.

This peak flow meter measures how well you push air out of your lungs.

El metro de flujo máximo mide su capacidad de expulsar aire de los pulmones.

The peak flow meter helps me see how well your treatment is working.

El metro de flujo máximo ayuda a evaluar la eficacia de su tratamiento.

Mechanical ventilation

Ventilación mecánica

You need to have a tube inserted into your windpipe to help you breathe.

Tenemos que introducirle un tubo hasta la tráquea para ayudarle a respirar.

The tube will be connected to a machine that helps you breathe.

El tubo se conectará a máquina que lo ayuda a respirar.

The machine is called a ventilator.

Esta máquina se llama ventilador mecánico.

You will not be able to talk while the tube is in place.

Ud. no podrá hablar mientras tenga colocado el tubo.

Nebulizer

Nebulizador

This is a nebulizer.

Éste es un nebulizador.

The nebulizer will deliver medication to your lungs to help you breathe.

El nebulizador le llevará medicamento a los pulmones para ayudarle a respirar.

Hold the mouthpiece in your mouth and breathe in the medication.

Sostenga la boquilla en su boca y aspire el medicamento.

Oxygen via a mask

Máscara de oxígeno

You need oxygen.

Ud. necesita oxígeno.

This is an oxygen mask.

Ésta es una máscara de oxígeno.

The mask fits over your nose and mouth. Oxygen flows through the mask.

La máscara se coloca sobre la nariz y la boca y el oxígeno fluye por la máscara.

Oxygen via nasal cannula

You need oxygen.

This is a nasal cannula.

The prongs go into your nose and oxygen flows through them.

Oxígeno suministrado por cánula nasal

Ud. necesita oxígeno.

Ésta es una cánula nasal.

Las puntas se ponen dentro de la nariz y el oxígeno pasa por ellas.

Pulse oximeter

This is a pulse oximeter.

A pulse oximeter lets us check the oxygen content of your blood.

I need to put a probe on your finger.

Oxímetro para medir el pulso

Éste es un oxímetro.

Un oxímetro del pulso nos permite observar el contenido de oxígeno en la sangre.

Necesito ponerle una sonda en el dedo.

Suctioning

I need to suction secretions from your breathing tube.

Suctioning your breathing tube will make you cough.

Succión

Tengo que aspirar secreciones de su tubo de respiración.

Succionar de su tubo de respiración lo hará toser.

Tracheostomy

You need a tracheostomy.

The surgeon will make an incision through your windpipe and insert a tube to help you breathe.

You will be given an anesthetic before this procedure.

I need to clean your tracheostomy.

I need to suction your tracheostomy.

Suctioning will make you cough.

Traqueotomía

Ud. necesita una traqueotomía.

El cirujano le hará una incisión quirúrgica por la tráquea y le insertará un tubo para ayudarle a respirar.

Se le dará anestesia antes de este procedimiento.

Tengo que limpiar su traqueotomía.

Tengo que aspirar su traqueotomía.

Esta succión le hará toser.

Specialty beds

Air-therapy bed

You need a special bed called an air-therapy bed.

This bed helps prevent skin breakdown.

This type of bed has air-filled compartments.

Cama para terapia respiratoria

Ud. necesita una cama especial que se llama cama para terapia respiratoria.

Evitará que su piel se lesione.

Este tipo de cama tiene compartimientos llenos de aire.

Clinitron therapy bed

You need to have a Clinitron therapy bed temporarily.

This bed will help prevent bedsores.

When you are in this bed, your bed will feel like you are in a waterbed.

Cama Terapéutica Clinitron

Ud. necesita provisionalmente una cama terapéutica Clinitron.

Esta cama prevendrá las úlceras de decúbito.

Cuando esté en esta cama, sentirá como si estuviera en una cama de agua.

Specimen collection equipment

Arterial blood gas analysis

I need to draw blood to check the oxygen in your blood.

You are going to feel a needle stick.

I need to apply pressure to stop the bleeding.

Análisis de gas de sangre arterial

Necesito sacarle sangre para controlar el nivel de oxigeno en sangre.

Ud. va a sentir un piquete de aguja.

Necesito aplicarle presión para detener la salida de sangre.

Blood glucose monitor

This blood glucose monitor measures your blood sugar.

I need to prick your finger to get a drop of blood.

Your blood sugar is _____.

Monitor de glucosa en sangre

Este monitor de glucosa en sangre se usa para medir el azúcar en la sangre.

Necesito pincharle el dedo para obtener una gota de sangre.

El nivel de azúcar en su sangre es _____.

I need to give you some insulin.

Tengo que darle insulina.

Urine specimen

Muestra de orina

I need a urine specimen.

Necesito una muestra de su orina.

You need to urinate into this specimen container.

Ud. tiene que orinar en este recipiente.

Venipuncture

Punción venosa

I need to draw a sample of your blood.

Necesito sacarle una muestra de sangre.

I am going to place a tourniquet on your arm. It will feel tight.

Le voy a poner un torniquete en el brazo. Lo sentirá ajustado.

You are going to feel a needle stick.

Ud. va a sentir un piquete de aguja.

I need to apply pressure to stop the bleeding.

Necesito aplicar presión para detener el sangrado.

Wound care equipment

Drainage bag

Saco de drenaje

I am going to put a bag over your drain.

Le voy a poner un saco sobre su drenaje.

Dressing

Vendaje

I need to change your dressing

Tengo que cambiarle su vendaje.

I need to wash out your wound.

Tengo que enjuagar su herida.

I am going to clean the area around your wound.

Voy a limpiar el área alrededor de su herida.

I am going to remove the tape; it may pull a bit.

Voy a quitarle la cinta adhesiva; le puede tirar un poco.

Montgomery straps

Bandas de Montgomery

These are Montgomery straps.

Éstas son bandas de Montgomery.

I am going to place these straps next to your wound to make it easier to change your dressing.

Voy a colocarlas en su herida para facilitar cambio de vendaje.

Whirlpool bath

You need to take a whirlpool bath to help your wound heal.

Wound packing

I am going to remove the packing from your wound.

I am going to replace your wound packing.

Let me know if you have any pain.

Wound care

This Unna boot will help keep pressure off your wound.

Piscina de hidromasaje

Ud. necesita un baño en una piscina de hidromasaje para ayudar a sanar su herida.

Cobertura de heridas

Voy a quitarle la cobertura de su herida.

Voy a cambiarle la cobertura de su herida.

Avíseme si le duele.

Cuidado de heridas

Esta venda elástica ayudará a evitar la presión sobre su herida.

6

Nutrition and diet therapy

Nutrition

Dietary habits

Do you eat three large meals or several small meals each day?

What have you eaten in the past 24 hours?

What have you eaten during the past three days?

Do you eat at fast-food restaurants?
– How often?
    Once per week?
    Two times per week?
    Every day?

What items do you usually order?
– Pancakes?
– Egg sandwiches?
– French fries?
– Hamburger?
– Cheeseburger?
– Fish?
– Salad?
– Tacos?
– Burritos?
– Chicken?

Dietary influences

Does your ethnic or cultural background affect what you eat?
– How?
    Do you eat only vegetables?
    Do you eat red meat?

Hábitos alimentarios

¿Come tres comidas grandes o varias comidas pequeñas al día?

¿Qué ha comido en las ultimas 24 horas?

¿Qué ha comido en los últimos tres días?

¿Come en restaurantes donde se compra comida rápida
– ¿Con qué frecuencia?
    ¿Una vez a la semana?
    ¿Dos veces a la semana?
    ¿Todos los días?

Por lo general, ¿qué platos pide?
– ¿Panqueques?
– ¿Sandwhiches de huevo?
– ¿Papas fritas?
– ¿Hamburguesa?
– ¿Hamburguesa con queso?
– ¿Pescado?
– ¿Ensalada?
– ¿Tacos?
– ¿Burritos?
– ¿Pollo?

Influencias en la dieta

¿Su origen étnico o cultural ejerce una influencia sobre su dieta?
– ¿Cómo?
    ¿Come sólo verduras?
    ¿Come carne roja?

Do you eat only chicken or fish?	¿Come sólo pollo o pescado?
Does your religion affect what you eat?	**¿Su religión afecta lo que Ud. come?**
– How?	– ¿Cómo?
Are there special days when you fast or do not eat food?	¿Ayuna o no come nada durante días especiales?
Do you not eat meat on Fridays?	¿No come carne los viernes?

Weight / Peso

Have you gained any weight recently?	**¿Ha aumentado de peso últimamente?**
– How much?	– ¿Cuánto?
Have you lost any weight recently?	**¿Ha bajado de peso últimamente?**
– How much?	– ¿Cuánto?

Daily menu / Menú diario

Which foods do you eat during the day?	**¿Qué come en el transcurso del día?**
Do you have any food allergies?	**¿Sufre de alguna alergia alimentaria?**
– What are they?	– ¿Cuáles son?
Are there foods that you believe you should not eat?	**¿Hay alimentos que Ud. sabe que no debiera comer?**
– What are these foods?	– ¿Cuáles son éstos?
Why do you believe you should not eat these foods?	**¿Por qué cree Ud. que no debiera comerlos?**
How do these foods affect you?	**¿Cómo le afectan estos alimentos?**

(See *Using a list of foods,* pages 56 and 57.)

Fluid intake / Toma de líquidos

How many servings do you drink each day of:	**¿Cuántas porciones de las siguientes bebidas toma Ud. al día?**
– coffee?	– ¿Café?
– tea?	– ¿Té?
– cola?	– ¿Gaseosas cola?
– cocoa?	– ¿Chocolate?
– water?	– ¿Agua?
How much liquid do you drink during the day?	**¿Cuánto líquido bebe Ud. al día?**

Teeth and gums

How do you take care of your teeth and gums?

Do you have tooth or gum problems that make it hard for you to eat?

Dientes y encías

¿Qué cuidado les da a sus dientes y las encías?

¿Tiene algún problema con los dientes o las encías que interfiera con su habilidad de comer?

Food preparation

Who does the food shopping in your home?

Do you have adequate storage and refrigeration?

Who prepares the meals in your home?

Where is your food prepared?

Do you eat alone or with others?

Preparación de comidas

¿Quién compra la comida en su casa

¿Tiene lugares adecuados de almacenamiento y refrigeración?

¿Quién prepara las comidas en su casa?

¿Dónde se preparan los alimentos?

¿Come Ud. solo(a) o con otras personas?

Special diets

Do you follow a special diet?
– What kind of diet?
    Diabetic diet?
    Gluten-free diet?
    High-fiber diet?

    High-protein diet?

    Lactose-free diet?
    Low-calorie diet?
    Low-carbohydrate diet?
    Low-cholesterol diet?
    Low-fat diet?
    Low-fiber diet?
    Low-protein diet?
    Low-sodium diet?

Who prescribed the diet?

How long have you been on the diet?

What is the reason for the diet?

Dietas especiales

¿Tiene Ud. una dieta especial?
– ¿Qué clase de dieta? ·
    ¿Dieta para diabéticos?
    ¿Dieta sin gluten?
    ¿Dieta con alto contenido de fibra?
    ¿Dieta con alto contenido de proteína?
    ¿Dieta sin lactosa?
    ¿Dieta baja en calorías?
    ¿Dieta baja en carbohidratos?
    ¿Dieta baja en colesterol?
    ¿Dieta baja en grasa?
    ¿Dieta baja en fibra?
    ¿Dieta baja en proteínas?
    ¿Dieta baja en sal?

¿Quién le recetó la dieta?

¿Hace cuánto tiempo que realiza esta dieta?

¿Cuál es la razón por la cual sigue esta dieta?

Using a list of foods

Ask your patient to look at this list of foods and point to those he is allergic to or must restrict from his diet. You can also use the words here to help him plan meals or adjust his diet to accommodate foods that he likes or dislikes.

Cómo usar una lista de comidas

Solicite a su paciente que lea esta lista de comidas y señale a cuál de ellas es alérgico o debe limitar en su dieta. También puede utilizar las palabras mencionadas aquí para ayudarle a planificar sus comidas o ajustar su dieta para acomodar las comidas que le gustan o que no le gusta.

Grains	**Granos**	Cherries	Cerezas
Corn bread	Pan de maíz	Grapefruit	Toronja, pomelo
Rice	Arroz		
Rye bread	Pan de centeno	Grapes	Uvas
Tortillas	Tortillas	Orange	Naranja
Wheat bread	Pan de trigo	Peach	Durazno, melocotón
White bread	Pan blanco		
		Pear	Pera
Dairy	**Lácteos**	Pineapple	Piña, ananá
Butter	Manteca	Strawberries	Fresas, frutillas
Cheese	Queso	Watermelon	Sandía
Eggs	Huevos		
Milk	Leche	**Vegetables and beans**	**Vegetales y frijoles**
Yogurt	Yogur	Baked beans	Frijoles horneados
Fruits	**Frutas**		
Apple	Manzana	Black beans	Frijoles negros
Banana	Plátano, banana	Broccoli	Brócoli
		Corn	Maíz
Cantaloupe	Melón cantalupo	Cucumbers	Pepinos

Sodium intake

Do you limit your salt intake?

– Why?

How much salt do you use, if any?

Ingesta de sodio

¿Limita Ud. la cantidad de sal que consume?
– ¿Por qué?

¿Cuánta sal usa Ud., si es que la usa?

Supplements

Do you supplement your diet with vitamins, calcium, protein, or other products?
– Which supplements do you use?

Suplementos

¿Complementa Ud. su dieta con vitaminas, calcio, proteínas u otros productos?
– ¿Qué suplementos consume?

Green beans	Ejotes, judías verdes (habichuelas)	Soda	Soda
		Tea	Té
Lettuce	Lechuga	**Meat**	**Carnes**
Onions	Cebollas	Beef	Carne de res
Peas	Guisantes, arvejas	Hamburger	Hamburguesa
		Pork	Puerco
Peppers	Pimientos	Ribs	Costillas
Pinto beans	Judías pintas		
Potatoes	Papas	**Fish**	**Pescado**
Red beans	Frijoles rojos	Flounder	Lenguado
Refried beans	Frijoles refritos	Salmon	Salmón
Spinach	Espinaca	Shrimp	Camarón
Tomatoes	Tomates	Tuna	Atún
Cereals	**Cereales**	**Poultry**	**Carne de ave**
Cold cereal	Cereal frío	Chicken	Pollo
Cream of wheat	Crema de trigo	Turkey	Pavo
Oatmeal	Harina de avena	**Snacks**	**Bocadillos**
		Cake	Pastel
Beverages	**Bebidas**	Chips	Papitas
Apple juice	Jugo de manzana	Cookies	Galletas dulces
		Crackers	Galletas saladas
Cranberry juice	Jugo de arándano	Ice cream	Helado
		Peanuts	Cacahuates
Coffee	Café	Pretzels	Pretzels
Grape juice	Jugo de uva		
Grapefruit juice	Jugo de toronja	**Condiments**	**Condimentos**
		Ketchup	Ketchup
Orange juice	Jugo de naranja	Mayonaise	Mayonesa
		Mustard	Mostaza
Pineapple juice	Jugo de piña		

– In what amounts?

Does your current problem affect your ability to cook and eat?

Is it hard for you to open cans or cut meat?

Food groups

Do you regularly eat foods from each of the five basic food groups?
– Grains?
– Vegetables?

– ¿En qué cantidades?

¿Su habilidad de cocinar y comer es afectada por su problema actual?

¿Tiene Ud. dificultad para abrir latas o cortar carne?

Grupos de comidas

¿Come habitualmente alimentos de cada uno de los cinco grupos alimentarios básicos?
– ¿Granos?
– ¿Vegetales?

– Fruits?
– Meats?
– Dairy products?
(See *My Pyramid*.)

– ¿Frutas?
– ¿Carnes?
– ¿Productos lácteos?

Diet therapy

Special diets

Your doctor has ordered a special diet for you.

This diet is called a:
– diabetic diet.
– gluten-free diet.
– high-fiber diet.

– high-protein diet.

– lactose-free diet.
– low-calorie diet.
– low-carbohydrate diet.
– low-cholesterol diet '
– low-fat diet.
– low-fiber diet.
– low-protein diet.
– low-sodium diet.

The doctor wants you to eat more (less) _____.

Too much _____ can make your _____ worse.

Eating more _____ can improve your _____.

The dietitian will speak with you about your _____ diet.

Dietas especiales

Su doctor ha recetado una dieta especial para Ud.

La dieta se llama:
– dieta para diabéticos.
– dieta sin gluten.
– dieta con alto contenido de fibra.
– dieta con alto contenido de proteínas.
– dieta sin lactosa.
– dieta baja en calorías.
– dieta baja en carbohidratos.
– dieta baja en colesterol.
– dieta baja en grasa.
– dieta baja en fibra.
– dieta baja en proteínas.
– dieta baja en sal.

El doctor quiere que Ud. coma más (menos) _____.

Demasiado(a) _____ puede empeorar su _____.

El comer más _____ puede mejorar su _____.

El/La dietista hablará con Ud. acerca de su dieta _____.

Sodium intake

You need to reduce the amount of salt in your diet.

Check labels for the amount of salt in foods you buy.

Avoid adding salt:
– while cooking your food.
– to your food at the table.

Ingetsa de sodio

Ud. necesita reducir el consumo de sal en su dieta.

Controle las etiquetas para ver la cantidad de sal que contienen las comidas que compra.

Evite añadir sal:
– cuando cocine su comida.
– a la comida en la mesa.

(Text continues on page 62.)

My Pyramid   Mi Pirámide

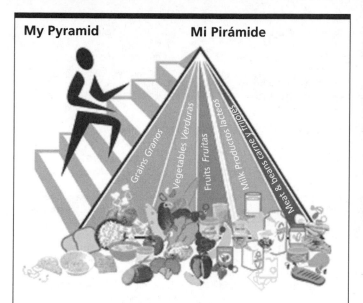

Grains
– Make half of your grains whole.
– Eat at least 3 oz of whole-grain cereals, breads, crackers, rice, or pasta every day.

– 1 oz is about 1 slice of bread, about 1 cup of breakfast cereal, or ½ cup of cooked rice, cereal, or pasta.

Vegetables
– Vary your vegetables.
– Eat more dark-green veggies such as broccoli, spinach, and other dark leafy greens.

– Eat more orange veggies such as carrots and sweet potatoes.

– Eat more dry beans and peas such as pinto beans, kidney beans, and lentils.

Granos
– Consuma la mitad en granos integrales.
– Consuma al menos 3 onzas de cereals, panes, galletas, arroz o pasta provenientes de granos intergrales todos los dias.
– Una onza es, aproximadamente, 1 rebanada de pan o ? taza de arroz, cereal o pasta cocidos.

Verduras
– Varíe las verduras.
– Consuma mayor cantidad de verdures de color verde oscuro como el brócoli, la espinaca y otras verdures de color verde oscuro.
– Cosuma mayor contidad de verdures de color naranja como zanahorias y batatas.
– Cosuma mayor cantidad de frijoles y guisantes secos como frijoles pinto, colorados y lentejas.

(continued)

My Pyramid (continued)
Fruits
– Focus on fruits
– Eat a variety of fruit.
– Choose fresh, frozen, canned, or dried fruit.
– Limit how much fruit juice you drink.

Milk
– Consume calcium-rich foods.

– Pick low-fat or fat-free when you choose milk, yogurt, and other milk products.

– If you don't or can't consume milk, choose lactose-free products or other calcium sources, such as fortified foods and beverages.

Meats and beans
– Go lean with protein.

– Choose low-fat or lean meats and poultry.
– Bake it, broil it, or grill it.

– Vary your protein routine; choose more fish, beans, peas, nuts, and seeds.

Food group recommendations
For a 2,000 calorie diet, you need the amounts below from each food group. To find the amounts that are right for you, go to *MyPyramid.gov.*

– Grains: Eat 6 oz every day.

– Vegetables: Eat 2½ cups every day.
– Fruits: Eat 2 cups every day.
– Milk: Get 3 cups every day; for kids ages 2 to 8, 2 cups.

Mi Pirámide (continuacíon)
Frutas
– Enfoque en las frutas.
– Consuma una variedad de frutas.
– Elija frutas frescas, congeladas, enlatadas o secas.
– No tome mucha cantidad de jugo de frutas.

Productos lácteos
– Coma alimentos ricos en calcio.

– Al elegir leche, opte por leche, yogur y otros productos lácteos descremados o bajos en contenido graso.
– En caso de que no consuma o no pueda leche, elija producots sin lactosa u otra fuente de calcio como alimentos y bebidas fortalecidos.

Carnes y frijoles
– Escoja proteinas bajas en grasas.
– Elija carnes y aves de bajo contenido graso o magras.
– Cocínelas al horno, a la parrilla o a la plancha.
– Varie la rutina de proteinas que consume; consuma mayor cantidad de pescado, frijoles, guisantes, nueces y semillas.

Recomendaciones solare grupos alimetarios
En una dieta de 2,000 calorías, necesita consumir las siguientes cantidades de cada grupos de alimentos. Para consultar las cantidades correctas para usted, visite MyPyramid.gov.
– Granos: Coma 6 onzas cada día.
– Verduras: Coma 2½ tazas cada día.
– Frutas: Coma 2 taza cada día.
– Productos lácteos: Coma 3 tazas cada día; para ninos edades 2-8, 2 tazas.

– Meat and beans: Eat 5½ oz every day.

Find your balance between food and physical activity

– Stay within your daily calorie needs.

– Be physically active for at least 30 minutes most days of the week.

– About 60 minutes a day of physical activity may be needed to prevent weight gain.

– For sustaining weight loss, at least 60 to 90 minutes a day of physical activity may be required.

– Children and teenagers should be physically active for 60 minutes every day or most days.

Know the limits on fats, sugars, and salt (sodium)

– Make the most of your fat sources from fish, nuts, and vegetable oils.

– Limit solid fats like butter, stick margarine, shortening, and lard as well as foods that contain these.

– Check the Nutrition Facts label to keep saturated fats, trans fats, and sodium low.

– Choose food and beverages low in added sugars. Added sugars contribute calories with few, if any, nutrients.

– Carnes y frijoles: Coma 5½ onzas cada día.

Encuentre el equilibrio entre lo que come y su actividad física

– Asegúrese de mantenerse dentro de sus necesidades calóricas diarias.

– Manténgase físicamente activo por lo menos durante 30 minutos la mayoria de los días de la semana.

– Es posible que necesite alrededor de 60 minutos diarios de actividad física para evitar subir de peso.

– Para mantener la pérdida de peso, se necesitan al menos entre 60 y 90 minutos diarios de actividad física

– Los ninos y adolescentes deberían estar fisicamente activos durante 60 minutos todos los dias o lay mayoría de los dias.

Conozca los límites de las grasas, los azúcares y la sal (sodio)

– Trate de que la mayor parte de su fuente de grasas provenga del pescado, las nueces y los aceites vegetales.

– Limite las grasas sólidas como la mantequilla, la margarina, a mantea vegetal y la manteca de cerdo, así como los alimentos que los contengan.

– Verifique las etiquetas de Datos Nutricionales para mantener bajo el nivel de grasas saturadas, grasas *trans* y sodio.

– Elija alimentos y bebidas con un nivel bajo de azúcares agregados. Los azucares agregados aportan calorias con pocos o ningún nutriente.

Adapted from U.S. Department of Agriculture. Center for Nutrition Policy and Promotion. (2005). MyPyramid Mini-Poster [Online]. Available: http://www.mypyramid.gov/downloads/miniposter.pdf [2006, September 5].

Use herbs or salt substitutes to add flavor to your food.

Use hierbas o sustitutos de sal para añadirle sabor a su comida.

Low-cholesterol

You need to reduce the amount of cholesterol in your diet.

Some foods that you should not eat are:
- butter
- shortening
- egg yolks
- biscuits
- cheese
- avocados
- bacon
- sausage
- hot dogs
- shellfish
- ice cream
- chocolate
- liver
- most red meat.

Bajo colesterol

Ud. necesita reducir la cantidad de colesterol en su dieta.

Algunos de los alimentos que Ud. no debe comer son:
- mantequilla
- grasa (manteca)
- yemas de huevo
- panecillos
- queso
- aguacate
- tocino
- salchicha
- perros calientes
- mariscos
- helado
- chocolate
- hígado
- la mayoría de la carne roja.

High-fiber

You need to add fiber to your diet.

Eating more fiber helps lower cholesterol and your risk of heart disease, colon cancer, and diabetes.

Eat fresh fruit and vegetables.
- High-fiber fruits include apples, oranges, and peaches.

- High-fiber vegetables include carrots, string beans, broccoli, and peas.

Eat whole grain breads, such as whole wheat and pumpernickel, and whole grain cereals, such as bran flakes, oat flakes, oatmeal, and shredded wheat.

Alto contenido de fibras

Ud. tiene que añadir fibra a su dieta.

El comer más fibra le ayudará a reducir el colesterol y el riesgo de contraer enfermedades del corazón, cáncer del colon y diabetes.

Coma fruta fresca y verduras.
- Algunas frutas con alto contenido de frita son las manzanas, naranjas y melocotones.
- Algunas verduras con alto contenido de frita son las zanahorias, ejotes, brócoli y guisantes (chícharos).

Coma pan integral, como pan de trigo entero y pan negro de centeno, y cereal de grano integral, como hojuelas de avena, harina de avena y trigo molido.

Eat dried peas and beans, such as lentils and navy, kidney, or pinto beans.

Add unprocessed bran to your food.

Remember to drink at least six 8-ounce glasses of water per day.

Coma guisantes secos y frijoles como lentejas, frijoles rojos, frijoles negros y frijoles pintos.

Añada salvado de trigo sin procesar a sus comidas.

No se olvide de tomar por lo menos seis vasos de ocho onzas de líquido al día.

7

Skin, hair, and nails

Current health problems

Hair loss

Have you noticed hair loss?

– Where?
– How long has this been happening?

Have you recently been exposed to:
– radiation?
– chemotherapy?
– hair chemicals?

– scalp infections?
    When?
    Did you receive treatment?
    How was your condition
      treated?

Have you recently been sick?

– What was your illness?
– How was it treated?

Nail problems

Have you noticed changes in your fingernails or toenails?
– What type of change?
    Breakage?
    Splitting?
    Discoloration?
    Other?

When did you first notice the problem?

Has the problem worsened or improved?

Pérdida de cabello

¿Ha notado pérdida de cabello en general o en ciertas partes?
– ¿Dónde?
– ¿Desde hace cuánto tiempo?

¿Ha estado expuesto recientemente a:
– radiación?
– quimioterapia?
– productos químicos para el cabello?
– infecciones del cuero cabelludo?
    ¿Cuándo?
    ¿Recibió tratamiento?
    ¿Cómo fue tratada la afección?

¿Ha estado enfermo recientemente?
– ¿Quál fue la enfermedad?
– ¿Qué tratamiento recibió?

Problemas de las uñas

¿Ha notado algún cambio en las uñas?
– ¿Qué tipo de cambio?
    ¿Se le quiebran?
    ¿Se le parten?
    ¿Decoloración?
    ¿Otra cosa?

¿Cuándo notó este problema por primera vez?

¿Ha empeorado o mejorado el problema?

Skin and hair
La piel y el cabello

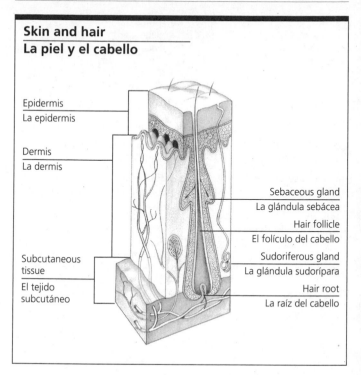

Epidermis
La epidermis

Dermis
La dermis

Sebaceous gland
La glándula sebácea

Hair follicle
El folículo del cabello

Subcutaneous
tissue

Sudoriferous gland
La glándula sudorípara

El tejido
subcutáneo

Hair root
La raíz del cabello

What makes the problem worse?	¿Qué es lo que empeora el problema?
What makes the problem better?	¿Qué es lo que alivia el problema?

Skin problems

Problemas de la piel

What bothers you most about your skin problem?	¿Qué aspecto de su problema de la piel le molesta más?
Where on your body did the skin problem begin?	¿En qué parte del cuerpo comenzó su problema de la piel?
When did you first notice the problem?	¿Cuándo se dió cuenta por primera vez de este problema?
Has the problem spread to other areas? – To what areas? – In what order?	¿Se le ha extendido el problema a otras partes? – ¿A qué zonas – ¿En qué orden?
How would you describe your skin problem? – Soreness?	¿Cómo describiría Ud. su problema de la piel? – ¿Dolor?

– Rash? | – ¿Erupción?
– Dryness? | – ¿Sequedad?
– Flaking? | – ¿Escamosa?
– Discoloration? | – ¿Decoloración?
– Itching? | – ¿Comezón (picazón)?
– Other? | – ¿Otra cosa?

How big is it? | **¿De qué tamaño es?**

What color is it? | **¿De qué color es?**

Do you have other symptoms? | **¿Tiene otros síntomas?**
– What are they? | – ¿Cuáles son?

Do you have any moles? | **¿Tiene lunares?**
– Have any new moles developed recently? | – ¿Le han salido lunares recientemente?
– Where? | – ¿Dónde?
– Have any of your moles changed in appearance, become larger, become painful, developed a discharge, or bled? | – ¿Han cambiado de apariencia algunos de sus lunares, han crecido, se han vuelto dolorosos, tienen secreción o han sangrado?
– What color are they? | – ¿De qué color son?
– Are they: | – Son:
    round? | ¿redondos?
    irregularly shaped? | ¿de forma irregular?
    raised? | ¿con relieve?
    flat? | ¿planos?

How does your skin feel? | **¿Qué sensaciones tiene en la piel?**

Have you noticed skin changes in other areas? | **¿Ha notado cambios en la piel en otras partes?**

Can you relate the skin problem to: | **¿Puede relacionar el problema de la piel con:**
– stress? | – estrés?
– contact with a particular substance? | – contacto con alguna sustancia en particular?
– change in your activities? | – cambio de actividades?

Does anything make the problem worse? | **¿Hay algo que agrava el problema?**
– Food? | – ¿Alimentos?
– Heat? | – ¿El calor?
– Cold? | – ¿El frío?
– Exercise? | – ¿El ejercicio?
– Sunlight? | – ¿La luz del sol?
– Stress? | – ¿El estrés?
– Pregnancy? | – ¿El embarazo?
– Menstruation? | – ¿La menstruación?

Does anything make the problem better? – What?	**¿Hay algo que le alivie el problema?** – ¿Qué?
Does the problem seem to be getting better?	**El problema, ¿parece estar mejorando?**

Have you used anything to make the problem better?
– What?
  Medications?
  Compresses?
  Lotions?
  Creams?
  Ointments?
	¿Ha consumido algo para resolver su problema?
	– ¿Qué?
	  ¿Medicamentos?
	  ¿Compresas?
	  ¿Lociones?
	  ¿Pomadas?
	  ¿Ungüentos?

Medical history

Have you had any fever, sickness or breathing or stomach problems? – When? – How was it treated?	**¿Ha tenido fiebre, malestar o problemas con la parte respiratoria o estomocales?** ¿Cuándo? ¿Qué tratamiento recibió?
Have you ever had anything like this before?	**¿Ha tenido alguna vez algo parecido?**
Have you had any allergic reactions to foods or other substances, such as make-up? – What caused it? – What reaction occurred?	**¿Ha tenido alguna reacción alérgica a alimentos u otras sustancias, tal como cosméticos?** – ¿Qué la provocó? – ¿Qué reacción tuvo?
Have you recently had any other illnesses, such as heart problems, muscle aches, or infections? – When? – How was the condition treated?	**¿Ha tenido recientemente cualquier otra enfermedad, tal como problemas del corazón, dolor de músculos o infecciones?** – ¿Cuándo? – ¿Qué tratamiento recibió la afección?

Family history

Has anyone in your family had a skin problem? – What was it? – When did it occur? – How was it treated?	**¿Ha tenido algún miembro de su familia un problema de piel?** – ¿Cuál fue? – ¿Cuándo ocurrió? – ¿Qué tratamiento recibió?

Has anyone in your family had an allergy?	**¿Hay alguien de su familia que haya tenido alguna alergia?**
– To what were they allergic?	– ¿Cuál fue?
– How was the allergy treated?	– ¿Qué tratamiento recibió?

Health patterns

Medications

Medicamentos

Do you take any medications?
- Prescription?
- Over-the-counter?
- Home remedies?
- Herbal preparations?
- Other?

¿Toma algún medicamento?
- ¿Con receta?
- ¿De venta libre?
- ¿Remedios caseros?
- ¿Preparados herbles?
- ¿Otro?

Which prescription medications do you take?
- How often do you take them?

¿Qué medicamentos con receta toma Ud.?
- ¿Con qué frecuencia los toma?

Which over-the-counter medications do you take?
- How often do you take them?

¿Qué medicamentos de venta libre toma?
- ¿Con qué frecuencia los toma?

Why do you take these medications?

¿Por qué toma estos medicamentos?

How much of each medication do you take?

¿Cuál es la dosis de cada uno de ellos?

How does each medication make you feel?

¿Cómo le hace sentirse cada uno de estos medicamentos?

Are you allergic to any medications?
- Which medications?
- What happens when you have an allergic reaction?

¿Es Ud. alérgico(a) a cualquier medicamento?
- ¿Qué medicamentos?
- ¿Qué ocurre cuando Ud. tiene una reacción alérgica?

Personal habits

Hábitos personales

Do you smoke or chew tobacco?

- What do you smoke?
    Cigarettes?
    Cigars?
    Pipe?
- How long have you smoked or chewed tobacco?
- How many cigarettes, cigars, or pipes of tobacco do you smoke each day?
- How much tobacco do you chew each day?

¿Fuma o masca tabaco?

- ¿Qué fuma?
    ¿Cigarrillos?
    ¿Cigarros (puros)?
    ¿Pipa?
- ¿Hace cuánto tiempo fuma o masca tabaco?
- ¿Cuántos cigarrillos, cigarros (puros) o pipas de tabaco fuma Ud. al día?
- ¿Cuánto tabaco masca Ud. al día?

– Did you ever stop?
  For how long did you stop?

  What made you decide to stop?
  What method did you use to stop?
  Do you remember why you started again?

Have you smoked or chewed tobacco in the past?
– If you do not use tobacco now, what influenced you to stop?

Do you drink alcoholic beverages?
– What type?
  Beer?
  Wine?
  Hard liquor?
– How often do you drink alcoholic beverages?
– How many drinks do you have in one day?

What do you think makes a person's skin healthy?

What do you do to try to keep your skin healthy?

What would you like to do for your skin but feel you cannot do?

What type of soap and skin creams or lotions do you use?
– How often do you use them?

What do you use when you wash your clothes?
– Do you use fabric softener?
– How do you dry your clothes?

Do you use gel or other styling products on your hair?
– What do you use?
– How often do you use these products?

How often do you shampoo?

– ¿Dejó de fumar alguna vez?
  ¿Cuánto tiempo estuvo sin fumar?
  ¿Por qué decidió dejar de fumar?
  ¿Qué método usó Ud.?

  ¿Recuerda por qué comenzó a fumar otra vez?

¿Ha fumado o mascado tabaco en el pasado?
– Si no consume tabaco actualmente, ¿qué fue lo que le influyó a dejar de fumar?

¿Toma bebidas alcohólicas?

– ¿Qué tipo?
  ¿Cerveza?
  ¿Vino?
  ¿Aguardiente?
– ¿Con qué frecuencia bebe?

– ¿Cuántos tragos toma en un día?

¿Qué piensa Ud. que causa que una persona tenga piel saludable?

¿Qué hace Ud. para conservar su piel saludable?

¿Qué quisiera hacer por su piel, pero no lo puede hacer?

¿Qué tipo de jabón o pomadas o lociones para el cutis usa Ud.?
– ¿Con qué frecuencia las usa?

¿Qué usa para lavar la ropa?

– ¿Usa suavizante de ropa?
– ¿Cómo seca la ropa?

¿Usa gel u otros productos de modelado del cabello?
– ¿Qué usa Ud.?
– ¿Con qué frecuencia usa estos productos?

¿Con qué frecuencia se lava Ud. el cabello?

– What kind of shampoo do you use?

– ¿Qué tipo de champú usa?

Do you use make-up or perfumes?

¿Usa maquillaje o perfumes?

– What types?

– ¿Qué tipos?

Do you shave with a blade or an electric razor?

¿Se rasura con navaja o con máquina de afeitar eléctrica?

Do you use a depilatory?

¿Usa un producto depilatorio?

Do you color your hair?

¿Se tiñe el cabello?

How do you trim your nails?

¿Cómo se corta las uñas?

Sleep patterns

Patrones de sueño

How many hours do you sleep each night?

¿Cuántas horas duerme por noche?

When you wake up, do you feel rested?

Cuando se despierta, ¿se siente bien descansado?

Has your sleep pattern changed recently?

¿Ha cambiado recientemente su patrón de sueño?

– How?

– ¿Cómo?

– Are you sleeping more or less than usual?

– ¿Duerme más o menos de lo habitual?

Has your skin problem caused you to lose sleep?

Su problema de piel, ¿ha hecho que duerma menos?

Activities

Actividades

Has your skin problem affected your daily activities?

¿Su problema de la piel ha afectado sus actividades diarias?

– How?

– ¿Cómo?

What are your recreational activities?

¿Cuáles son sus actividades recreativas?

Do these activities expose you to:

¿Estas actividades lo exponen (a):

– sun or other light?

– al sol u otra luz?

– chemicals or other kinds of poisons?

– productos químicos u otros tipos de tóxicos?

– animals?

– animales?

– outdoors?

– al aire libre?

– foreign travel?

– viajes al extranjero?

Nutrition

Nutrición

Describe what you typically eat during the day.

Describa lo que come habitualmente durante el día.

How much water do you drink each day?

¿Cuánta agua bebe or dia?

Sexual patterns

Has your skin problem interfered with your sex life?
– How?

Environment

How much time do you spend outdoors?

How often is your skin exposed to the sun?

Do you use sunblock?
– How often?
– What strength?

Have you ever had severe sunburn?
– When?

Does your work expose you to:
– sun or other types of light?
– chemicals or other poisons?

– animals?
– outdoors?
– foreign travel?

Patrones sexuales

¿Su problema de la piel ha interferido con su sexualidad?
– ¿Cómo?

Entorno

¿Cuánto tiempo pasa al aire lebre?

¿Cuán a menudo expone su piel al sol?

¿Usa pantalla solar?
– ¿Con cuánta frecuencia?
– ¿De qué factor?

¿Alguna vez ha sufrido quemaduras de sol graves?
– ¿Cuándo?

¿Su trabajo le expone:
– al sol u otra luz?
– a productos químicos u otras toxinas?
– a animales?
– al aire libre?
– a viajes al extranjero?

Psychosocial considerations

Coping skills

How does the affected area of your skin look to you?

How does your skin problem make you feel?

What concerns you about your skin problem and its treatment?

Have you recently had any stress or emotional problems, such as an unplanned job change or relationship issues?

– How have you handled these problems?

Habilidad de sobrellevar los problemas

¿Cómo ve el área afectada de la piel?

¿Cómo le hace sentirse su problema de la piel?

¿Qué preocupaciones tiene Ud. con relación a su problema de la piel y su tratamiento?

¿Ha tenido Ud. recientemente algún problema de estrés o emocional, tal como un cambio de trabajo imprevisto o un problema afectivo?

– ¿Cómo ha manejado estos problemas?

Roles

How has your skin problem affected your relationships with others?

How do you feel about going out socially?

Has your skin problem interfered with your role as a spouse (or student, parent, or other) or with your sex life?

Roles

¿Cómo le ha afectado su problema de la piel en sus relaciones conlos demás?

¿Cómo se siente al salir socialmente?

¿Su problema de la piel ha interferido con su papel de esposo(a) (o de estudiante, de padre, de madre, u otro) o con su vida sexual?

Responsibilities

What kind of work do you do now?

What kind of work have you done in the past?

Has your skin problem affected your job?
– How?

Responsabilidades

¿Qué tipo de trabajo realiza actualmente?

¿Qué tipo de trabajo ha realizado anteriormente?

Su problema de piel, ¿ha afectado su trabajo?
– Cómo?

Developmental considerations

For the pediatric patient

Is the infant breast-fed or formula-fed?
– What formula do you use?

Has the infant had any skin problems related to a particular formula or food added to the diet?

Has the infant had any diaper rashes that did not clear up by using over-the-counter skin preparations?

What kind of diapers do you use?
– How do you wash cloth diapers?

Para el (la) paciente de pediatría

¿Le da Ud. de mamar o lo alimenta con fórmula?
– ¿Qué fórmula usa?

¿Ha tenido el(la) niño(a) algún problema de la piel relacionado con una fórmula en particular o algún alimento que se le haya añadido a su dieta?

¿Ha tenido el(la) niño(a) alguna erupción de la piel que no se le haya quitado fácilmente con alguna preparación para la piel de venta libre?

¿Qué clase de pañales usa Ud.?

– ¿Cómo lava Ud. los pañales de tela?

How often do you bathe the infant?

¿Con qué frecuencia baña Ud. al niño (la niña)?

What soaps, creams, or lotions do you use on the infant's skin?

¿Qué jabones, cremas o lociones usa Ud. en la piel de su criatura?

How do you dress the infant in hot weather? In cold weather?

¿Cómo viste Ud. a la criatura cuando hace calor y cuando hace frío?

Does the child go to day care or nursery school?

¿Va la criatura a una guardería de niños?

Do you have an older child who is in kindergarten or elementary school?

¿Tiene Ud. un hijo mayor en el jardín de infancia o en la escuela primaria?

Do you have pets in your home?
– What type of pets?

¿Tiene Ud. animales en casa?
– ¿Qué clase de animales?

Does the child sleep with stuffed animals?

¿Duerme la criatura con animales de juguete?

Has the child been scratching the scalp?

¿Se rasca la criatura el cuero cabelludo?

Does the skin or scalp scale in circular patterns?

¿La piel o el cuero cabelludo se escama en forma circular?

Has the child lost an unusual amount of hair?
– When did this start?

¿Ha perdido la criatura una cantidad inusual de cabello?
– ¿Cuándo empezó a ocurrir esta pérdida?

Has the child been pulling his or her hair?

¿El niño o la niña se jala el cabello?

Has the child ever had warts?

¿Ha tenido la criatura verrugas alguna vez?

– On what part of the body?
– How were they treated?

– ¿En qué parte del cuerpo?
– ¿Qué tratamiento se les dió?

Does the child play where he might come into contact with bugs, weeds, or bushes?
– How often does he play there?

¿El niño, ¿juega donde puede estar en contacto con bichos, hierbas, o arbustos?
– ¿Con qué frecuencia juega allí?

For the adolescent patient

Para la paciente adolescente

What do you usually eat each day?

¿Qué come Ud. normalmente a diario?

Have you had any bad cuts or scrapes from falls or other accidents?
– How long did it take for them to heal?

¿Ha tenido algún corte grave o raspaduras a causa de caídas u otros accidentes?
– ¿Cuánto tiempo tardaron en sanar?

Do you bite your nails?

¿Se muerde las uñas?

Do you twirl your hair or play with it?

¿Se enrosca o juega de otra manera con el cabello?

Does your face, upper back, or chest ever break out in pimples?

¿Le salen alguna vez erupciones en la cara, la parte superior de la espalda o en el pecho?

For the pregnant patient

Para la paciente embarazada

Have you noticed changes in your skin during your pregnancy?
– What kind of change?
– Where did you first notice it?

– When did you first notice it?

¿Ha notado Ud. algún cambio en la piel durante su embarazo?

– ¿Qué tipo de cambio?
– ¿Dónde lo observó Ud. por primera vez?
– Cuándo lo observó por primera vez?

For the elderly patient

Para el (la) paciente anciano(a)

Has your skin changed as you have aged?
– How?
– How do you feel about the skin changes you have noticed?

¿Le ha cambiado la piel al envejecer?
– ¿Cómo?
– ¿Qué piensa acerca de los cambios de la piel que Ud. ha notado?

Have you had any recent falls or other accidents?

¿Se ha caído Ud. recientemente o ha tenido otros accidentes?

Have you noticed any difference in how wounds or sores heal?
– What kind of difference?

¿Ha notado Ud. alguna diferencia en la manera en que sanan sus heridas o llagas?
– ¿Qué tipo de diferencia?

Do temperature changes, touch, or pressure affect your skin?

– How?

¿Su piel es afectada por los cambios de temperatura o cuando la toca o aplica presión sobre ella?
– ¿Cómo?

8

Head and neck

Current health problems

Difficulty swallowing

Do you have any trouble swallowing?
- How would you describe this problem?
- How long have you had it?

Do you have problems with anything you eat and drink?
- What things cause you difficulty?
- Is there any time of day when the problem is worse?

Do you have any trouble chewing?
- How would you describe this problem?
- Does it bother you all the time or only when you eat or drink?
- When did it start?

Facial swelling

Is your face swollen?

- When did you first notice the swelling?

- Have you noticed a change in the swelling?
    Is the swelling worse?

    Is the swelling better?

- Does anything make the swelling better?

Dificultad para tragar

¿Tiene Ud. alguna dificultad para tragar?
- ¿Cómo la describiría Ud.?

- ¿Hace cuánto que tiene este problema?

¿Tiene problemas con alguna cosa que coma o beba?
- ¿Qué cosas le causan dificultad?

- El problema, ¿empeora en algún momento del dia?

¿Tiene Ud. alguna dificultad al mascar?
- ¿Cómo describiría Ud. esta dificultad?
- ¿Ocurre todo el tiempo o sólo cuando come o bebe?
- ¿Cuándo empezó a ocurrir?

Inflamación facial

¿Tiene Ud. la cara inflamada/hinchada?
- ¿Cuándo notó Ud. la inflamación/hinchazón por primera vez?
- ¿Ha notado Ud. algún cambio en la inflamación?
    ¿Ha empeorado la inflamación?
    ¿Ha mejorado la inflamación?
- ¿Hay algo que mejore la inflamación?

Mouth
La boca

Posterior pillar
El pilar posterior

Stensen's duct
El conducto
de Stensen

Anterior
pillar

El pilar
anterior

Oropharynx

La orofaringe

Sulcus
terminalis

El surco
terminal

Sublingual
gland ducts

El conducto de la
glándula sublingual

Vestibule

El vestíbulo

Gingivae

Las encías

Frenulum of upper lip
El frenillo del labio
superior

Hard palate
El paladar duro

Soft palate
El paladar
blando

Uvula
La úvula

Tonsil
La amígdala

Tongue
La lengua

Wharton's
duct

El conducto
de Wharton

Frenulum
of lower lip

El frenillo del
labio inferior

- Does anything make the
  swelling worse?

**Is there swelling in any other
areas, such as:**
- The jaws?
- Behind the ear?
    When did it occur?

**Do you have any other signs or
symptoms when you have
swelling, such as:**
- pain?

- ¿Hay algo que empeore la inflamación?

**¿Tiene Ud. inflamación en otras
partes, como:**
- la mandíbula?
- detrás de la oreja?
    ¿Cuándo ocurrió?

**¿Tiene Ud. otros síntomas que
acompañan la inflamación, tal
como:**
- dolor?

– tenderness?
– redness?
– warmth?
– impaired movement?
  Where?

– sensibilidad?
– enrojecimiento?
– entibiamiento de la zona?
– menor movimiento?
  ¿Dónde?

Headaches

Do you have headaches?
– How long do they last?
– How often do you get headaches?
  Frequently?
  Rarely?

Do the headaches seem to follow a pattern?
– What kind of pattern?

When do you usually get a headache?
– Early morning?
– During the day?
– At night?
– Certain times of the month?
– With certain types of weather?

What kind of pain accompanies the headache?
– Sharp or stabbing?

– Dull ache?
– Throbbing?
– Pressure?
– Other?

Where do you feel the pain?
– Across your forehead?
– Behind your eyes?
– Along your temples?
– In the back of your head?

Do any other signs or symptoms accompany the headache?
– What are they?
  Nausea?
  Vomiting?
  Stiff neck?
  Blurred vision?
  Sensitivity to light?
  Other?

What do you do to relieve the headaches?

Dolores de cabeza

¿Tiene Ud. dolores de cabeza?
– ¿Cuánto tiempo duran?
– ¿Con qué frecuencia tiene dolores de cabeza?
  ¿Frecuentemente?
  ¿Casi nunca?

¿Siguen algún patrón sus dolores de cabeza?
– ¿Qué clase de norma?

¿Por lo general cuándo tiene dolores de cabeza?
– ¿En la mañana temprano?
– ¿Durante el día?
– ¿En la noche?
– ¿Durante cierta época del mes?
– ¿Con cierto tipo de clima?

¿Qué clase de dolor acompaña el dolor de cabeza?
– ¿Agudo o punzante, como una cuchillada?
– ¿Dolor sordo?
– ¿Palpitante?
– ¿Presión?
– ¿Otra clase?

¿Dónde siente Ud. el dolor?
– ¿A través de la frente?
– ¿Atrás de los ojos?
– ¿Por las sienes?
– ¿Atrás de la cabeza?

¿Hay otros síntomas que acompañan el dolor de cabeza?
– ¿Cuáles son?
  ¿Náuseas?
  ¿Vómito?
  ¿Cuello tenso?
  ¿Visión borrosa?
  ¿Sensibilidad a la luz?
  ¿Otro?

¿Qué hace Ud. para mitigar el dolor de cabeza?

Hoarseness

Do you have any hoarseness?
– When did you first notice it?

Have you noticed changes in the sound of your voice?
– What kind of change?

What makes it better?

What makes it worse?

Nasal discharge

Do you have any discharge from your nose?
– When did you first notice it?

– When does it occur?
    All the time?
    In the morning?
    At night?
    Other?
– Does it seem to follow a pattern?
    What kind of pattern?

How would you describe the discharge?
– Thick?
– Thin?
– Watery?
– Like pus?

What color is the discharge?
– Clear?
– White?
– Yellow?
– Green?
– Red?
– Other?

Do you have any allergies?
– To what are you allergic?

Do you have any other signs or symptoms, such as:
– fever?
– headache?
– cough?
– wheezing?
– other?

Ronquera

¿Tiene Ud. ronquera?
– ¿Cuándo la notó por primera vez?

¿Ha notado Ud. algún cambio en el sonido de su voz?
– ¿Qué clase de cambio?

¿Qué mejora la ronquera

¿Qué empeora la ronquera

Secreción nasal

¿Tiene Ud. secreción nasal?

– ¿Cuándo la notó por primera vez?
– ¿Cuándo ocurre?
    ¿Todo el tiempo?
    ¿Por la mañana?
    ¿En la noche?
    ¿Otro?
– ¿Parece seguir un patrón?

    ¿Qué tipo de patrón?

¿Cómo describiría Ud. la secreción?
– ¿Espesa?
– ¿No densa?
– ¿Acuosa?
– ¿Parecida a pus?

¿De qué color es la secreción?
– ¿Claro?
– ¿Blanco?
– ¿Amarillo?
– ¿Verde?
– ¿Roja?
– ¿Otro?

¿Tiene Ud. alergias?
– ¿A qué?

¿Tiene Ud. otros síntomas, tales como:
– fiebre?
– dolor de cabeza?
– tos?
– respiración jadeante?
– otro?

Has the discharge improved or worsened since it started?

¿Ha mejorado o empeorado la secreción desde que comenzó?

What aggravates it?

¿Qué es lo que la agrava?

What relieves it?

¿Con qué se mejora?

Neck stiffness

Cuello tenso

Is your neck stiff?

¿Tiene Ud. el cuello tenso?

When did the stiffness begin?

¿Cuándo empezó la tensión?

How would you describe the stiffness?
– Constant?
– Intermittent?

¿Cómo la describiría Ud.?

– ¿Constante?
– ¿Intermitente?

Does the stiffness occur at any specific time?
– When?
    Early morning?
    During the day?
    After activities?

    At night?
    While you are sleeping?

¿Ocurre la tensión en un momento en particular?
– ¿Cuándo?
    ¿Temprano por la mañana?
    ¿Durante el día?
    ¿Después de hacer actividades?
    ¿En la noche?
    ¿Mientras Ud. duerme?

Is the stiffness worse than it used to be?

¿Ha aumentado la tensión desde que comenzó?

Do you have pain as well as stiffness?
– What is the pain like?

¿La tensión produce dolor?

– ¿Cómo es el dolor?

Do you sometimes hear a grating sound or feel a grating sensation, as if your bones are scraping together?

¿Hay veces que Ud. oye un sonido áspero o siente una sensación chirriante, como si los huesos se rasparan uno con el otro?

What have you tried to reduce the stiffness?
– What makes it better?
– What makes it worse?

¿Qué métodos ha empleado Ud. para reducir la tensión?
– ¿Qué la mejora?
– ¿Qué la empeora?

Nosebleed

Hemorragia nasal

Do you have nosebleeds?
– How often?
– How long have you been having nosebleeds?

¿Tiene Ud. hemorragia nasal?
– ¿Con qué frecuencia?
– ¿Cuánto tiempo hace que tiene hemorragias?

Do you notice that the nosebleeds happen at a particular time?
– When?

¿Ha observado Ud. si las hemorragias se producen en un momento particular?
– ¿Cuándo?

How long do the nosebleeds last?
- Less than a minute?
- A few minutes?
- Longer?

What do you usually do to stop the nosebleeds?

Are your nosebleeds worse than they used to be?

¿Cuánto tiempo duran las hemorragias?
- ¿Menos de un minuto?
- ¿Unos cuantos minutos?
- ¿Más tiempo?

¿Qué hace Ud. para detener la hemorragia?

Las hemorragias nasales, ¿son peores que antes?

Ulcers

Úlceras

Do you have any ulcers?
- Where?
  In your nose?
  In your mouth?
  On your tongue?
  On your lips?
  Other?

¿Tiene Ud. úlceras?
- ¿Dónde?
  ¿En la nariz?
  ¿En la boca?
  ¿En la lengua?
  ¿En los labios?
  ¿En otra parte?

How would you describe them?
- Soft?
- Hard?
- Crusty?
- Moist?

¿Cómo las describiría Ud.?
- ¿Blandas?
- ¿Duras?
- ¿Costrosas?
- ¿Húmedas?

How long have you had them?

- Do they clear up and come back?

¿Hace cuánto tiempo que Ud. las tiene?
- ¿Desaparecen y luego vuelven a aparecer?

Do you notice that the ulcers appear at any particular time?

- When?

¿Ha notado Ud. si las úlceras aparencen en un momento en particular?
- ¿Cuándo?

Do the ulcers make it hard for you to eat or drink?
- How?

Sus úlceras, ¿le molestan al comer o?
- ¿Cómo?

What makes them better?

¿Qué las mejora?

What makes them worse?

¿Qué las empeora?

Medical history

Have you ever had any allergies that made it hard for you to breathe and gave you the feeling that your throat was closing?
- When did these symptoms usually occur?

¿Ha tenido Ud. alguna vez alguna alergia que le causó dificultad para respirar y que le dió la sensación de que la garganta se le cerraba?
- ¿En qué ocasiones ocurrían típicamente estos síntomas?

– How did you deal with them?

– How were they treated?

Have you ever had a neck injury or had trouble moving your neck in any direction?

– What was the injury?

– When did it occur?

– What helped relieve it?

Have you ever had neck surgery?

– When?

– For what reason?

Have you ever had:

– head trauma?

– skull surgery?

– jaw surgery?

– facial fractures?

  When?

– What treatment did you receive?

Do you have a history of sinus infections or tenderness?

– When did it start?

– How was it treated?

Have you had headaches or tightness in the neck or jaw?

– What makes it better?

  Relaxation?

  Exercise?

  Massage?

– Is the headache or neck or jaw tightness related to:

  lack of sleep?

  missed meals?

  stress?

– ¿Cómo los manejó?

– ¿Qué tratamiento tuvieron?

¿Ha tenido Ud. alguna vez una lesión en el cuello o dificultad mover el cuello en cualquier dirección?

– ¿Cuál?

– ¿Cuándo ocurrió?

– ¿Qué le alivió?

¿Ha tenido Ud. cirugía en el cuello?

– ¿Cuándo?

– ¿Por qué razón?

¿Ha tenido Ud. alguna vez:

– trauma de la cabeza?

– cirugía del cráneo?

– cirugía de la mandíbula?

– fracturas de la cara?

  ¿Cuándo?

– ¿Qué tratamiendo recibió?

Tiene Ud. un historial de infecciones o sensibilidad de los senos frontales?

– ¿Cuándo empezó?

– ¿Qué tratamiento se le dió?

¿Ha sufrido Ud. de dolores de cabeza o tensión del cuello o de la mandíbula?

– ¿Qué hace que se mejore?

  ¿Relajación?

  ¿Ejercicio?

  ¿Masaje?

– El dolor de cabeza o del cuello o la tensión de la mandíbula se relaciona con:

  ¿La falta de sueño?

  ¿El hecho saltearse comidas?

  ¿El estrés?

Family history

Have any of your family members had a neurologic disease?

– What disease?

– Which relative?

– How was it treated?

¿Ha tenido algún miembro de su familia una enfermedad neurológica?

– ¿Qué enfermedad?

– ¿Qué pariente?

– ¿Qué tratamiento recibió?

Have any of your family members had:
- high blood pressure?
- stroke?
- heart disease?
- headaches?
- arthritis?
    When?
    How was it treated?

¿Hay algún miembro de su familia que haya tenido:
- presión sanguínea alta?
- ataque apopléjico?
- enfermedad cardiaca?
- dolores de cabeza?
- artritis?
    ¿Cuándo?
    ¿Qué tratamiento se le dió?

Health patterns

Medications

Do you take any medications?
- Prescription?
- Over-the-counter?
- Home remedies?
- Herbal preparations?
- Other?

Which prescription drugs do you take?
- How often do you take them?

Which over-the-counter medications do you take?
- How often do you take them?

Why do you take these medications?

How much of the medication do you take each time?

How does each medication make you feel?

Are you allergic to any medications?
- Which medications?
- What happens when you have an allergic reaction?

Medicamentos

¿Toma Ud. medicamentos?
- ¿De receta?
- ¿De venta libre?
- ¿Remedios caseros?
- ¿Preparados herbalas?
- ¿Otros?

¿Qué medicamentos con receta toma Ud.?
- ¿Con qué frecuencia los toma?

¿Qué medicamentos de venta libre toma?
- ¿Con qué frecuencia los toma?

¿Por qué toma Ud. estos medicamentos?

¿Qué dósis de medicamento toma en cada ingesta?

¿Cómo le hace sentirse cada uno de estos medicamentos?

¿Es Ud. alérgico(a) a cualquier medicamento?
- ¿Qué medicamentos?
- ¿Qué pasa cuando Ud. tiene una reacción alérgica?

Personal habits

Do you smoke or chew tobacco?
- What do you smoke?
    Cigarettes?
    Cigars?
    Pipe?
- How long have you smoked or chewed tobacco?

Hábitos personales

¿Fuma Ud. o masca tabaco?

- ¿Qué fuma Ud.?
    ¿Cigarrillos?
    ¿Cigarros (puros)?
    ¿Pipa?
- ¿Hace cuánto tiempo que fuma o masca Ud. tabaco?

– How many cigarettes, cigars, or pipes of tobacco do you smoke per day?

– How much tobacco do you chew per day?

– Did you ever stop?

What made you decide to stop?

For how long did you stop?

What method did you use to stop?

Do you remember why you started again?

If you do not use tobacco now, have you smoked or chewed tobacco in the past?

Do you drink alcoholic beverages?

– What type?

Beer?

Wine?

Hard liquor?

– How often do you drink alcoholic beverages?

– How many drinks do you have in one day?

Spread over how much time?

Do you grind your teeth?

How often do you brush and floss your teeth?

When was the last time you went to the dentist?

– What were the results of the examination?

Do you wear a seat belt when you are in an automobile?

Sleep patterns

How many hours do you sleep each night?

When you wake up, do you feel rested?

– ¿Cuántos cigarrillos, cigarros (puros) o pipas de tabaco fuma Ud. al día?

– ¿Cuánto tabaco masca Ud. al día?

– ¿Alguna vez dejó Ud. de fumar o mascar?

¿Qué lo hizo decidirse a deja de fumar?

¿Cuánto tiempo duró?

¿Qué método usó Ud. para dejar de fumar o mascarlo?

¿Recuerda Ud. porque volvió al hábito otra vez?

Si no consume tabaco actualmente, ¿ha fumado o mascado tabaco en el pasado?

¿Toma Ud. bebidas alcohólicas?

– ¿Qué clase?

¿Cerveza?

¿Vino?

¿Aguardiente?

– ¿Con qué frecuencia toma bebidas alcohólicas?

– ¿Cuántos tragos toma en un día?

¿Durante cuánto tiempo?

¿Cruje Ud. sus dientes?

¿Con qué frecuencia se lava Ud. los dientes o usa hilo dental?

¿Cuándo fue la última vez que fue al dentista?

– ¿Cuáles fueron los resultados del examen dental?

¿Usa Ud. cinturón de seguridad cuando va en automóvil?

Patrones de sueño

¿Cuántas horas duerme por noche?

Cuando se despierta, ¿se siente bien descansado?

Has your head or neck problem interfered with your sleep pattern?
– How?

Su problema en la cabeza o el cuello, ¿ha interferido con su patrón de sueño?
– ¿Cómo?

Activities

Actividades

Has your head or neck problem interfered with your normal activities?
– How?

¿Su problema de la cabeza o del cuello ha interferido con sus actividades cotidianas?
– ¿Cómo?

Do you do any exercises to help with your problem?
– What exercises do you do?

¿Hace Ud. algún ejercicio para mejorar su problema?
– ¿Qué ejercicios realiza?

Do you play any sports that require you to wear a helmet?
– Which sports?
– How often do you play these sports?

¿Participa Ud. en algún deporte que exija el uso de casco?
– ¿Qué deportes?
– ¿Con qué frecuencia participa Ud. en estos deportes?

Nutrition

Nutrición

Has your head or neck problem made it hard for you to eat or drink?
– How?

¿Su problema de la cabeza o del cuello le dificulta la ingesta de bebidas o comidas?
– ¿Cómo?

What foods are hard for you to eat?

¿Con qué clase de alimentos tiene Ud. dificultad?

What foods are easy for you to eat?

¿Qué alimentos puede Ud. comer con facilidad?

Sexual patterns

Hábitos sexuales

Has your head or neck problem affected your sex life?

– How?

¿Ha interferido su problema de la cabeza o del cuello con sus actividades sexuales?
– ¿Cómo?

Environment

Entorno

Do weather changes seem to make the problem better or worse?
– How?

¿Le parece que los cambios climáticos mejoran o empeoran el problema
– ¿Cómo?

Does the problem worsen in cold or damp weather?

¿Se empeora el problema con el frío o con el tiempo húmedo?

Psychosocial considerations

Coping skills

Do you feel any stress because of your current problem?

What do you do to cope with stress?

Habilidad de sobrellevar un problema

¿Siente Ud. estrés a causa de su problema actual?

¿Qué medidas toma Ud. rutinariamente para hacer frente al estrés?

Roles

Does your head or neck problem affect the way you feel about yourself? The way you get along with your family?
– How?

Roles

¿Su problema de la cabeza o del cuello afecta la manera que Ud. se siente consigo mismo(a) o en su relación con su familia?
– ¿Cómo?

Responsibilities

Has your head or neck problem affected your ability to work?

– How?

Does your job require long hours of sitting, such as at a computer?

– How long do you sit?

Does your job put you at risk for head injury?

– Do you wear a hard hat?

Responsabilidades

Su problema en la cabeza o el cuello, ¿ha afectado su capacidad de trabajar?
– ¿Cómo?

¿Su trabajo le exige estar sentado(a) por muchas horas, por ejemplo, delante de una computadora?
– ¿Cuánto tiempo?

¿Su trabajo lo expone al riesgo de sufrir una herida en la cabeza?
– ¿Usa Ud. casco?

Developmental considerations

For the pediatric patient

Is your drinking water treated with fluoride?
– Does the child take fluoride tablets?

Does the child use a pacifier or suck his or her thumb?
– When did the child begin teething?

Para el (la) paciente de pediatría

¿Está el agua potable tratada con fluoruro?
– ¿Toma el niño (la niña) tabletas de fluoruro?

¿Usa la criatura un chupete o se chupa el dedo?
– ¿Cuándo comenzó la dentición del niño (la niña)?

– Does the child have tonsils?
When were they removed?
Why were they removed?

– ¿Tiene la criatura amígdalas?
¿Cuándo se las sacaron?
¿Por qué se las sacaron?

For the pregnant patient

Para la paciente embarazada

Have you noticed any head or neck problems during your pregnancy?
– What kind?

¿Ha notado algún problema en la cabeza o el cuelo durante su embarazo?
– ¿De qué tipo?

For the elderly patient

Para el (la) paciente anciano(a)

Do you wear dentures?

¿Tiene Ud. dentadura postiza?

Are they:
– upper?
– lower?
– both?

Son:
– ¿superiores?
– ¿inferiores?
– ¿ambas?

How long have you worn them?

¿Hace cuánto tiempo que la tiene?

How well do they fit?

¿Le queda bie?

Do they cause any pain or discomfort?

¿Le molesta o le causa dolor?

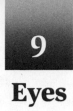

9

Eyes

Current health problems

Blurred vision

Do you have blurred vision?
– When did you first notice it?

– How long have you had it?

– Do you have it all the time?

Is the blurred vision associated with any activity, such as:
– sitting?
– standing?
– walking?
– changing positions?
– other?

Do you have any other signs or symptoms, such as:
– headache?
– dizziness?
– nausea?
– fainting?

Do you have any discharge or drainage from your eyes?
– How often?
– How much?
– What color is the discharge?

Does anything else occur with the blurred vision?
– Spots?
– Floaters?
– Halos around lights?
  Was this a sudden change or has it occurred for a while?

  How long?

Visión borrosa

¿Tiene Ud. visión borrosa?
– ¿Cuándo la notó Ud. por primera vez?

– ¿Hace cuánto tiempo que la tiene?

– ¿La tiene constantemente?

¿Se relaciona esto con cualquier actividad, tal como:
– estar sentado(a)?
– estar parado(a)?
– caminar?
– cambiar de posición?
– otra?

¿Tiene Ud. otros síntomas, tal como:
– dolor de cabeza?
– mareo?
– náuseas?
– desmayos?

¿Tiene alguna secreción en los ojos?
– ¿Con cuánta frecuencia?
– ¿Cuánta cantidad?
– ¿De qué color es la secreción?

La visión borrosa ¿trae aparejado algo más?
– ¿Manchas?
– ¿Círculos?
– ¿Luces con halos?
  ¿Fue éste un cambio súbito o lo ha tenido Ud. por algún tiempo?
  ¿Cuánto tiempo?

Does anything make it worse?

– What?

Does anything make it better?
– What?

¿Hay algo que agrave el problema?
– ¿Qué?

¿Hay algo que la alivie?
– ¿Qué?

Vision changes

Cambios en la visión

Do you have any problems seeing?

– What?

   Seeing objects that are far
      away?
   Seeing close objects?
   Other?

¿Tiene problemas de visión?

– ¿Qué problemas?
   ¿Ver objetos a distancia?

   ¿Ver objetos de cerca?
   ¿Otro?

Describe your problem.

Describa su problema.

Have you noticed a change in your vision?
– What change have you noticed?
– When did you first notice the
   change?

¿Ha notado Ud. algún cambio en su vista?
– ¿Qué cambio ha notado?
– ¿Cuándo notó Ud. este cambio
   por primera vez?

Do you wear glasses or contact lenses?
– How long have you worn them?

– Why do you wear them?

¿Usa anteojos o lentes de contacto?
– ¿Hace cuánto tiempo que los
   usa?
– ¿Por qué los usa?

Are your contact lenses hard or soft?

Sus lentes de contacto, ¿son duros o blandos?

How often do you wear glasses or contact lenses?
– All the time?
– For certain activities, such as:

   Reading?
   Close work?
   Driving?
   Other?

¿Con qué frecuencia usa los anteojos o los lentes de contacto?
– ¿Todo el tiempo?
– Para ciertas actividades, tales
   como:
   ¿Leer?
   ¿Trabajo minucioso?
   ¿Conducir?
   ¿Otro?

Did you ever stop wearing the glasses or contact lenses?

– Why?
– When did you stop?

¿Alguna vez dejó Ud. de usar los anteojos o los lentes de contacto?
– ¿Por qué?
– ¿Cuándo dejó Ud. de usarlos?

Eye
El ojo

Sclera
La esclerótica

Choroid layer
La capa coroides

Iris
El iris

Cornea
La córnea

Anterior
chamber
(filled with
aqueous
humor)
La cámara
anterior (llena
de humor
acuoso)

Conjunctiva
(bulbar)
La conjuntiva
(bulbar)

Canal of Schlemm
El conducto
de Schlemm

Retina
La retina

Central retinal artery
and vein
La arteria
y la vena
central retinal

Optic nerve
El nervio óptico

Vitreous humor
El humor vítreo

Ciliary body
El cuerpo ciliar

Lens
El lente

Posterior chamber
(filled with
aqueous humor)
La cámara posterior (llena
de humor acuoso)

Pupil
La pupila

Medical history

When was your last eye examination?
– What were the results?

Are your eyes often infected or inflamed?

– How often?
– How is the problem treated?

Have you ever had eye surgery?
– When?
– For what reason?
– What kind of surgery?

¿Cuándo tuvo Ud. su último examen de vista?
– ¿Cuáles fueron los resultados?

¿Sufre frecuentemente infecciones o inflamación de los ojos?
– ¿Con qué frecuencia?
– ¿Qué tratamiento recibe?

¿Ha tenido cirugía ocular?
– ¿Cuándo?
– ¿Por qué razón?
– ¿Qué clase de cirugía?

Have you ever had an eye injury?	**¿Ha tenido Ud. alguna vez una lesión en el ojo?**
– What kind of injury?	– ¿Qué clase de lesión?
– When did it happen?	– ¿Cuándo la tuvo?
– How was it treated?	– ¿Qué tratamiento recibió?
Have you ever had an eye infection?	**¿Tuvo alguna vez una infección ocular?**
– When?	– ¿Cuándo?
– How was it treated?	– ¿Cómo fue tratada?
Do you often have sties?	**¿Le salen orzuelos con frecuencia?**
– How often?	– ¿Con qué frecuencia?
– How are they treated?	– ¿Qué tratamiento se les da?
Do you have a history of high blood pressure or diabetes?	**¿Tiene Ud. un historial de presión sanguínea alta o de diabetes?**

Family history

Has anyone in your family ever been treated for:	**¿Hay algún miembro de su familia que haya tenido alguno de los siguientes problemas?**
– cataracts?	– ¿Cataratas?
– glaucoma?	– ¿Glaucoma?
– blindness?	– ¿Ceguera?
Who had the condition?	¿Quién fue?
How was it treated?	¿Qué tratamiento recibió?
Does anyone in your family have another eye problem?	**¿Hay algún miembro de su familia que tenga otro problema ocular?**
Does anyone in your family wear glasses or contact lenses?	**¿Hay algún miembro de su familia que use anteojos o lentes de contacto?**
– Who wears them?	– ¿Quién los usa?
– How long has he or she worn them?	– ¿Hace cuánto tiempo que los usa?
– Why does he or she wear them?	– ¿Por qué los usa?

Health patterns

Medications

Do you take any medications?	**¿Toma Ud. medicamentos?**
– Prescription?	– ¿Con receta?
– Over-the-counter?	– ¿De venta libre?
– Home remedies?	– ¿Remedios caseros?
– Herbal preparations?	– ¿Preparados herbales?
– Other?	– ¿Otro?

Medicamentos

Which prescription medications do you take?
– How often do you take them?

Which over-the-counter medications do you take?
– How often do you take them?

Why do you take these medications?

How much of each medication do you take?

How does each medication make you feel?

Are you allergic to any medications?
– Which medications?
– What happens when you have an allergic reaction?

¿Qué medicamentos con receta toma Ud.?
– ¿Con qué frecuencia los toma?

¿Qué medicamentos de venta libre toma?
– ¿Con qué frecuencia los toma?

¿Por qué toma Ud. estos medicamentos?

¿Qué dosis toma Ud. de cada uno?

¿Cómo le hace sentirse cada uno de estos medicamentos?

¿Es Ud. alérgica(o) a algún medicamento?
– ¿A cuál o cuáles?
– ¿Qué pasa cuando Ud. tiene una reacción alérgica?

Personal habits

Do you smoke or chew tobacco?
– What do you smoke?
  Cigarettes?
  Cigars?
  Pipe?
– How long have you smoked or chewed tobacco?
– How many cigarettes, cigars, or pipes of tobacco do you smoke per day?
– How much tobacco do you chew per day?
– Did you ever stop?
  For how long?
  What made you decide to stop?
  What method did you use to stop?

  Do you remember why you started again?

If you do not use tobacco now, have you smoked or chewed tobacco in the past?

Hábitos personales

¿Fuma Ud. o masca tabaco?
– ¿Qué fuma?
  ¿Cigarrillos?
  ¿Cigarros (puros)?
  ¿Pipa?
– ¿Hace cuánto tiempo que Ud. fuma o masca tabaco?
– ¿Cuántos cigarrillos, cigarros (puros) o pipas de tabaco fuma Ud. al día?
– ¿Cuánto tabaco masca al día?

– ¿Dejó Ud. el hábito alguna vez?
  ¿Por cuánto tiempo?
  ¿Qué hizo que se decidiera a dejar de fumar?
  ¿Qué método usó Ud. para dejar de fumar o mascar tabaco?
  ¿Recuerda Ud. por qué volvió a mascar o fumar otra vez?

Si actualmente no usa tabaco, ¿ha Ud. fumado o mascado tabaco en el pasado?

Do you drink alcoholic beverages?

– What type?
    Beer?
    Wine?
    Hard liquor?
– How often do you drink alcoholic beverages?
– How many drinks do you have in one day?
    Spread over how much time?

¿Toma Ud. bebidas alcohólicas?

– ¿Qué tipo?
    ¿Cerveza?
    ¿Vino?
    ¿Aguardiente?
– ¿Con qué frecuencia bebe bebidas alcohólicas?
– ¿Cuántos tragos toma en un día?
    ¿Durante cuánto tiempo?

Sleep patterns

How many hours of sleep do you get each night?

When you wake up, do you feel rested?

Does your eye problem affect your sleep?

Patrones de sueño

¿Cuántas horas duerme por noche?

Cuando se despierta, ¿se siente bien descansado?

Su problema en el ojo, ¿le afecta el sueño?

Activities

Do you play any sports?

What sports do you play?

Do you wear goggles when you play this sport?

Does your vision problem affect your social activities?
– How much?

Actividades

¿Participa algún deporte?

¿Qué deporte(s) practica?

¿Se pone Ud. anteojos protectores cuando hace deporte?

Su problema de visión, ¿restringe sus actividades sociales?
– ¿Hasta qué punto?

Nutrition

Describe what you usually eat each day.

Are you on a special diet?

How much water do you drink each day?

Nutrición

Describa lo que come normalmente por dia.

¿Tiene una dieta especial?

¿Cuánta agua bebe por dia?

Sexual patterns

Has your eye problem affected your usual sex life?
– How?

Patrones sexuales

Su problema en el ojo, ¿ha afectado su vida sexual habitual?
– ¿Cómo?

Environment

Does the air where you work or live contain anything that causes you eye problems, such as:
– cigarette smoke?
– chemicals?
– glues?
– formaldehyde insulation?
    What eye problems do you notice?

Does your occupation require close use of your eyes, such as long-term reading or prolonged use of a computer monitor?

Do you wear goggles when working with power tools, chain saws, or table saws?

Do you have any allergies, such as a pollen allergy?

Do your eyes itch?
– When?

Entorno

¿El ambiente donde Ud. trabaja o vive contiene algo que cause problemas en los ojos?

– ¿Humo de cigarrillos?
– ¿Productos químicos?
– ¿Pegamento, cola?
– ¿Aislamiento de formaldehído?
    ¿Qué problemas ha notado?

¿Su trabajo requiere que use mucho la vista, como leer o usar un monitor de computadora por mucho tiempo?

¿Usa Ud. anteojos protectores cuando trabaja con herramientas mecánicas, motosierras o sierras de mesa?

¿Tiene alergias, como alergia al polen?

¿Le pican los ojos?
– ¿Cuándo?

Psychosocial considerations

Coping skills

Do you feel stress because of your current problem?

What do you do to cope with stress?

Habilidad de sobrellevar un problema

Su problema actual, ¿le genera estrés?

¿Qué hace para hacerle frente al estrés?

Roles

How does wearing glasses or contact lenses make you feel about yourself?

Is wearing glasses or contact lenses a problem for you?

Roles

¿Cómo se siente Ud. al usar anteojos o lentes de contacto?

¿Le molesta usar anteojos o lentes de contacto?

Responsibilities

Does your health insurance cover the cost of eye examinations and lenses?

Responsabilidades

¿Su seguro médico cubre exámenes de vista y lentes?

Do vision problems make it difficult for you to do what you have to do at home or at work?	¿Sus problemas de visión le causan dificultad para cumplir con sus obligaciones en casa o en el trabajo?

Developmental considerations

For the pediatric patient	**Para el (la) paciente de pediatría**
Does the infant look at you or other objects?	¿La criatura mira fijamente a Ud. o a otros objetos?
Does the infant blink at bright lights or quick, nearby movements?	La criatura, ¿parpadea al ver luces brillantes o movimientos rápidos de objetos cercanos?
Do the child's eyes ever look crossed?	¿Hay veces que la criatura tiene bizquera?
Do the child's eyes ever move in different directions?	¿Hay ocasiones cuando los dos ojos se mueven en diferentes direcciones?
– Which directions?	– ¿En qué direcciones?
Does the child often rub the eyes?	¿La criatura se frota los ojos con frecuencia?
Does the child have any allergies?	El niño (la niña), ¿tiene alergias?
Does the child have any drainage from the eyes?	El niño (la niña), ¿tiene secreción ocular?
– How often?	– ¿Con cuánta frecuencia?
– How much?	– ¿Cuánta cantidad?
– What color is it?	– ¿De qué color?
Does the child squint a lot?	¿El niño (la niña) mira con frecuencia con los ojos entrecerrados?
Does the child often bump into objects or have difficulty picking up objects?	¿Se da el niño (la niña) golpes contra objetos con frecuencia o tiene dificultad en recoger objetos?
Does the child sit close to the television at home?	¿Se sienta el niño (la niña) muy cerca de la televisión?
How is the child doing in school?	¿Cómo le va al niño (la niña) en el colegio?
Does the child have to sit at the front of the classroom to see the chalkboard?	¿Se tiene que sentar la criatura en la parte delantera de la clase para poder ver la pizarra?

For the pregnant patient

Have you had any eye problems during your pregnancy?

Para la paciente embarazada

¿Ha tenido algún problema en los ojos durante su embarazo?

For the elderly patient

Do your eyes feel dry?

Do you have trouble seeing to the side but no trouble seeing what is in front of you?

Do you have problems with glare?

Do you have any problems telling one color from another?

Do you have difficulty seeing at night?
– What helps you see at night?

Para el (la) paciente anciano(a)

¿Siente secos los ojos?

¿Tiene Ud. dificultad para ver de costado pero no de frente?

¿Le molesta la luz brillante?

¿Tiene problemas para distinguir los colores?

¿Tiene Ud. dificultad para ver de noche?
– ¿Qué lo ayuda a ver de noche?

10

Ears

Current health problems

<table>
<tr><td>

Hearing changes

Have you recently noticed a change in your hearing?

– When did you first notice it?

Did you have any other medical problems when you first noticed the change?

Is the change only in one ear?
– Which ear?

Did the change come on suddenly?
– When?

When does the change in hearing occur?
– With all sounds?
– High-pitched sounds only?
– Low-pitched sounds only?

Is the change always present?
– When does it occur?

How would you describe the change?
– Muffling?
– Ringing?
– Crackling?
– Other?

Do you have any other symptoms, such as:
– Pain?
– Ringing in your ears?
– Headache?
– Pressure?
– Dizziness?

</td><td>

Cambios en la audición

¿Ha notado Ud. últimamente un cambio en su capacidad auditiva?

– ¿Cuándo lo notó Ud. por primera vez?

¿Tenía algún otro problema médico cuando notó el cambio por primera vez?

El cambio, ¿es sólo en un oído?
– ¿Qué oído?

¿Fue súbito este cambio?

– ¿Cuándo?

¿Cuándo ocurre el cambio en la audición?
– ¿Con todos los sonidos?
– ¿Sólo con sonidos agudos?
– ¿Sólo con sonidos graves?

El cambio, ¿ocurre siempre?
– ¿Cuándo ocurre?

¿Cómo describiría Ud. el cambio?
– ¿Sordo?
– ¿Zumbido?
– ¿Crujiente?
– ¿Otro?

¿Tiene Ud. otros síntomas, tal como:
– dolor?
– zumbido?
– dolor de cabeza?
– presión?
– mareo?

</td></tr>
</table>

External ear
El oído externo

Bony ear canal
El huesecillo del canal auditivo

Cartilaginous ear canal
El canal auditivo cartilaginoso

External auditory canal
El canal auditivo externo

Entrance to ear canal
La entrada al canal auditivo

Helix
El hélice

Antihelix
El anthélice

Concha
La concha

Lobule
El lóbulo

Mastoid process
El proceso mastoides

What makes it better?

What makes it worse?

Have you noticed any drainage from your ear?
– How much?
– How often does it occur?

– What color is it?

Tinnitus

Have you noticed ringing in your ears?
– When did you first notice it?

Is the ringing in only one ear?

¿Qué es lo que lo agrava?

¿Qué es lo que lo alivia?

¿Ha notado alguna secreción de su oído?
– ¿Cuánta cantidad?
– ¿Con cuánta frecuencia se produce?

– ¿De qué color es?

Tinnitus (Zumbido)

¿Ha notado Ud. un zumbido en los oídos?
– ¿Cuándo lo notó por primera vez?

¿Es el zumbido sólo en un oído?

Middle ear and inner ear
El oído medio y el oído interno

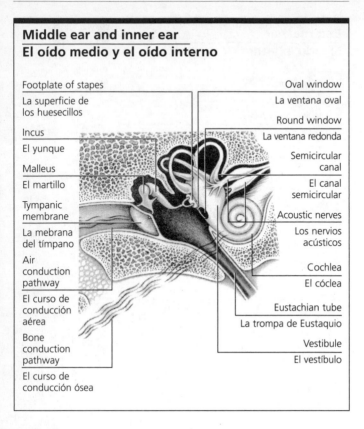

Footplate of stapes	Oval window
La superficie de los huesecillos	La ventana oval
	Round window
Incus	La ventana redonda
El yunque	
Malleus	Semicircular canal
El martillo	El canal semicircular
Tympanic membrane	Acoustic nerves
La mebrana del tímpano	Los nervios acústicos
Air conduction pathway	Cochlea
El curso de conducción aérea	El cóclea
	Eustachian tube
Bone conduction pathway	La trompa de Eustaquio
El curso de conducción ósea	Vestibule
	El vestíbulo

– Which ear?

Did the ringing begin suddenly?
– When?

Does the ringing in your ears occur all the time?
– How often does it occur?
– How long does it last?
– Is there anything that seems to occur before the ringing starts? What?

What makes the ringing better?

What makes the ringing worse?

Do you have any other symptoms when you hear the ringing?
– What?

– ¿En qué oído?

¿ Se produjo el zumbido de repente?
– ¿Cuándo?

¿Tiene Ud. el zumbido todo el tiempo?
– ¿Con qué frecuencia le ocurre?
– ¿Cuánto tiempo le dura?
– ¿Ocurre algo antes de comenzar el zumbido?
¿Qué?

¿Qué agrava el zumbido?

¿Qué alivia el zumbido?

¿Va acompañado este zumbido con otros síntomas?

– ¿Cuáles?

Medical history

When was your last time you had your ears examined?

¿Cuándo le examinaron por última vez los oídos?

When was your last hearing test?
– What were the results?

¿Cuándo fue su último examen de audición?
– ¿Cuáles fueron los resultados?

How do you routinely care for your ears?
– Do you use cotton swabs?

¿Cómo cuida Ud. habitualmente sus oídos?
– ¿Usa hisopos de algodón?

Do you wear a hearing aid?
– In which ear?
– Do you wear it all the time?
– How long have you worn it?

– Why did you get it?
– Does it help you hear better?

¿Usa Ud. un audífono?
– ¿En qué oído?
– ¿Se lo pone Ud. todo el tiempo?
– ¿Hace cuánto tiempo que lo usa?
– ¿Por qué lo compró?
– ¿Lo ayuda a oir mejor?

Have you ever had trouble with earwax?
– When?
– How was it treated?

¿Ha tenido problemas con la cerilla de los oídos?
– ¿Cuándo?
– ¿Qué tratamiento recibió?

Have you ever had an ear injury?
– When?
– What type of injury?
– How was it treated?

¿Ha tenido Ud. alguna vez una lesión en el oído?
– ¿Cuándo?
– ¿Qué tipo de lesión?
– ¿Qué tratamiento se le dió?

Have you ever had a foreign body in your ear?
– When?
– How was it treated?

¿Ha tenido Ud. alguna vez un cuerpo extraño en el oído?
– ¿Cuándo?
– ¿Qué tratamiento se le dió?

Do you have a lot of ear infections?
– How often do you get them?
– How long do they last?
– How are they treated?

¿Sufre Ud. de frecuentes infecciones del oído?
– ¿Con qué frecuencia?
– ¿Cuánto tiempo le duran?
– ¿Qué tratamiento se les ha dado?

Did you have a lot of ear infections when you were a child?
– How were they treated?

¿Tuvo muchas infecciones de oído durante la infancia?
– ¿Cómo fueron tratadas?

Did you ever have ear surgery?
– When?
– Why?

¿Ha sido operado de los oídos?
– ¿Cuándo?
– ¿Por qué?

Have you ever had tubes in your ears?
– When?

¿Alguna vez tuvo tubos en los oídos?
– ¿Cuándo?

Have you ever had drainage from your ears?
– When?
– How much?
– What color?
– How was it treated?

¿Ha tenido secrecions en los oídos?
– ¿Cuándo?
– ¿Cuánto?
– ¿De qué color?
– ¿Qué tratamiento se les dió?

Have you ever had problems with:

– Balance?
– Dizziness?
– Nausea?
– Vertigo?
    When?
    How was it treated?

¿Ha tenido Ud. alguna vez algunos de los siguientes problemas?
– pérdida del equilibrio?
– mareo?
– náuseas
– vértigo?
    ¿Cuándo?
    ¿Qué tratamiento se le dió?

Family history

Has anyone in your family ever had a hearing problem?

– Who?
– When did it occur?
– What kind of problem was it?
– How was it treated?

¿Hay algún miembro de su familia que haya tenido problemas de audición?
– ¿Quién fue?
– ¿Cuándo ocurrió esto?
– ¿Qué tipo de problema fue?
– ¿Qué tratamiento se le dió?

Health patterns

Medications

Do you take any medications?
– Prescription?
– Over-the-counter?
– Home remedies?
– Herbal preparations?
– Other?

Medicamentos

¿Toma Ud. medicamentos?
– ¿Con receta?
– ¿De venta libre?
– ¿Remedios caseros?
– ¿Preparados herbales?
– ¿Otro?

Which prescription drugs do you take?
– How often do you take them?

¿Qué medicamentos de receta toma Ud.?
– ¿Con qué frecuencia los toma Ud.?

Which over-the-counter medications do you take?
– How often do you take them?

¿Qué medicamentos de venta libre toma?
– ¿Con qué frecuencia los toma?

Why do you take these medications?

¿¿Por qué toma Ud. estos medicamentos?

How much of each medication do you take?

¿Qué dosis toma Ud. de cada medicamento?

How often do you take each medication?

¿Con qué frecuencia toma cada medicamento?

How does each medication make you feel?

¿Cómo le hace sentirse cada uno de estos medicamentos?

Are you allergic to any medications?
– Which medications?
– What happens when you have an allergic reaction?

¿Es Ud. alérgico(a) a algún medicamento?
– ¿A qué medicamentos?
– ¿Qué pasa cuando Ud. tiene una reacción alérgica?

Have you been taking any prescription medications, over-the-counter medications, or home remedies for your ears?
– What?
– How often do you use them?

¿Toma Ud. actualmente medicamentos con receta, medicamentos de venta libre o remedios caseros para el oído?
– ¿Cuál (cuáles)?
– ¿Con qué frecuencia?

Personal habits

Hábitos personales

Do you smoke or chew tobacco?
– What do you smoke?
  Cigarettes?
  Cigars?
  Pipe?
– How long have you smoked or chewed tobacco?
– How many cigarettes, cigars, or pipes of tobacco do you smoke per day?
– How much tobacco do you chew per day?
– Did you ever stop?

  For how long?
  What made you decide to stop?
  What method did you use to stop?
– Do you remember why you started again?

¿Fuma o masca Ud. tabaco?
– ¿Qué fuma Ud.?
  ¿Cigarrillos?
  ¿Cigarros (puros)?
  ¿Pipa?
– ¿Hace cuánto tiempo que Ud. fuma o masca tabaco?
– ¿Cuántos cigarrillos, cigarros (puros) o pipas de tabaco fuma Ud. al día?
– ¿Cuánto tabaco masca Ud. al día?
– ¿Ha dejado Ud. el hábito alguna vez?
  ¿Por cuánto tiempo lo dejó?
  ¿Qué lo hizo decidirse a dejar de fumar?
  ¿Qué método usó Ud. para dejarlo?
– ¿Recuerda Ud. por qué volvió a mascar o fumar otra vez?

If you do not use tobacco now, have you smoked or chewed tobacco in the past?

Si actualmente no usa tabaco, ¿ha Ud. fumado o mascado tabaco en el pasado?

Do you drink alcoholic beverages?
– What type?
  Beer?
  Wine?
  Hard liquor?

¿Toma Ud. bebidas alcohólicas?
– ¿Qué tipo?
  ¿Cerveza?
  ¿Vino?
  ¿Aguardiente?

– How often do you drink alcoholic beverages?
– How many drinks do you have in one day?
   Spread over how much time?

– ¿Con qué frecuencia bebe bebidas alcohólicas?
– ¿Cuántos tragos toma en un día?
   ¿Repartidas en cuánto tiempo?

Sleep patterns

How many hours of sleep do you get each night?

When you wake up, do you feel rested?

Has your ear problem affected your sleep pattern?

Patrones de sueño

¿Cuántas horas duerme por noche?

¿Cuando se despierta, ¿se siente biend descansado?

Su problema del oído, ¿ha afectado su patrón de sueño?

Activities

Does your hearing difficulty interfere with your daily activities?
– How?

Do you listen to loud music or turn up the television volume?

– How often?
– For how long each time?

Did you listen to loud music or go to concerts when you were younger?

Actividades

¿La dificultad auditiva interfiere en su vida cotidiana?

– ¿Cómo?

¿Escucha la música demasiado alta o pone Ud. la televisión más fuerte?
– ¿Con qué frecuencia?
– ¿Por cuánto tiempo cada vez?

¿Escuchaba música a alto volumen o iba a conciertos cuando era más joven?

Nutrition

Describe what you usually eat each day.

Are you on a special diet?
– What kind of diet?

Nutrición

Describa lo que generalmente come cada dia.

¿Tiene una dieta especial?
– ¿Qué tipo de dieta?

Sexual patterns

Has your ear problem affected your usual sexual activity?

– How?

Patrones sexuales

Su problema del oído, ¿ha afectado su actividad sexual habitual?
– ¿Cómo?

Environment

Do you spend time aroud equipment, such as heavy machinery, airguns, or airplanes?

Entorno

¿Está Ud. alrededor de equipos ruidosos, tales como maquinaria pesada, pistolas de aire o aviones?

– How long are you exposed to these noises each day?

– ¿Por cuánto tiempo al día está Ud. expuesto a ellos?

– Do you wear protective ear coverings when you are exposed to loud noises?

– ¿Usa protectores para el oído cuando Ud. está expuesto(a) a ellos?

Psychosocial considerations

Coping skills

Do you feel any stress because of your current problem?

What do you do to cope with stress?

Habilidad de sobrellevar problemas

¿Siente estrés a raíz de su problema actual?

¿Qué hace para lidiar con el estrés

Roles

Has your hearing difficulty changed the way you feel about yourself?

– How?

Roles

¿Su dificultad auditiva ha afectado la manera en que Ud. se siente respecto de usted mismo(a)?
– ¿Cómo?

Responsibilities

Does your hearing difficulty interfere with your daily work?
– How?

Does your hearing difficulty affect the way you get along with other people?
– How?

Responsabilidades

¿Su dificultad auditiva interfiere en su trabajo diario?
– ¿Cómo?

¿Su dificultad auditiva afecta sus relaciones con otras personas?
– ¿Cómo?

Developmental considerations

For the pediatric patient

Does the infant respond to loud or unusual noises?

Does the infant babble?

Does the toddler rely on gestures and not even try to make sounds?

Is the toddler speaking appropriately for his or her age?

Para el (la) paciente de pediatria

¿Responde el (la) infante(a) a ruidos fuertes o extraños?

¿Balbucea el (la) infante(a)?

¿El (la) pequeño(a) depende de ademanes y no trata de responder con sonidos

¿Habla el (la) pequeño(a) adecuadamente para su edad?

Have you noticed the child tugging at either ear?
– Which ear?

¿Ha notado Ud. si la criatura se jala una oreja?
– ¿Qué oreja?

Have you noticed any coordination problems?
– What?
– When did you first notice these problems?

¿Ha notado Ud. problemas de coordinación?
– ¿Cuáles?
– ¿Cuándo notó Ud. el problema por primera vez?

Has the child had any ear problem?
– What?
– When?
– How was it treated?

¿Ha tenido la criatura problemas en el oído?
– ¿Cuáles?
– ¿Cuándo?
– ¿Qué tratamiento se le dió?

Has the child been taking any medications?
– What?
– When?

La criatura, ¿ha estado tomando medicamentos?
– ¿Cuáles?
– ¿Cuándo?

For the pregnant patient

Para la paciente embarazada

Have you noticed any ear problems during your pregnancy?

¿Ha notado algún problema en el oído durante su embarazo?

For the elderly patient

Para el (la) paciente anciano(a)

Do you need to have people repeat things when they are talking to you?

¿Necesita que le repitan las cosas cuando le hablan?

Do you need to turn up the volume when you watch television?

¿Necesita subir el volumen al ver televisión?

11

Respiratory system

Current health problems

Chest pain

Do you have chest pain?
– Is it constant?
– Is it intermittent?
– Where do you feel the pain?

What activities produce the pain?

Does the pain occur when you breathe normally or when you take deep breaths?

What makes the pain better?

What makes the pain worse?

Confusion

Do you ever feel confused, restless, or faint?
– When does the feeling occur?
– How long does the feeling last?
– What makes it better?
– What makes it worse?

Cough

Do you have a cough?
– What does it sound like?
   Dry?
   Hacking?
   Barking?
   Congested?
– Does it usually occur at a certain time of day?
   When?
– What makes it better?
– What makes it worse?

Do you cough up sputum?

Dolor de pecho

¿Tiene Ud. dolor de pecho?
– ¿Es constante?
– ¿Es intermitente?
– ¿Dónde se localiza el dolor?

¿Qué actividad o actividades producen el dolor?

El dolor, ¿se produce cuando respira normalmente o cuando respira profundamente?

¿Qué alivia el dolor?

¿Qué intensifica el dolor?

Confusión

¿Alguna vez siente Ud. confusión, desasosiego o mareos?
– ¿Cuándo ocurre esto?
– ¿Cuánto tiempo dura?
– ¿Qué alivia la sensación?
– ¿Qué intensifica la sensación?

Tos

¿Tiene Ud. tos?
– ¿Qué sonido tiene?
   ¿Seco?
   ¿Aspero?
   ¿A tos perruna?
   ¿A congestión?
– ¿Por lo general, ocurre a cierta hora del día?
   ¿Cuándo?
– ¿Qué la alivia?
– ¿Qué la empeora?

¿Expectora Ud.?

Respiratory system
El sistema respiratorio

Choana	La coana
Sphenoid sinus	El seno esfenoidal
Nasopharynx	La nasofaringe
Oropharynx	La orofaringe
Laryngopharynx	La laringofaringe
Esophagus	El esófago
Trachea	La tráquea
Carina	La carina
Mediastinum	El mediastino
Hilum	El hilio
Left primary (mainstream)	El bronquio principal de la bronchus izquierda
Inferior nasal concha	La concha nasal inferior
Middle nasal concha	La concha nasal media
Superior nasal concha	La concha nasal superior
Frontal sinus	El seno frontal
Naris	Los nares
Soft palate	El paladar blando
Oral cavity	La cavidad bucal
Epiglottis	El epiglotis
Left secondary (lobar) Bronchus	El bronquio lobar de la izquierda
Bronchiole	El bronquiolo
Alveolus	El alvéolo
Thyroid cartilage	El cartílago tiroides

- How much sputum do you cough up each day?
- What color is it?
- How does it smell?
- Is it thick or thin?
- What time of day do you cough up the most sputum?
    Morning?
    Night?
    After meals?

- ¿Cuánto expectora Ud. al día?
- ¿De qué color es?
- ¿Qué olor tiene?
- ¿Es el esputo denso o claro?
- ¿A qué hora del día expectora Ud. más?
    ¿Por la mañana?
    ¿Por la noche?
    ¿Después de las comidas?

Fluid retention

Do your ankles swell?

Do you have trouble breathing at night?

What makes your symptoms better?

What makes your symptoms worse?

Have you gained any weight recently?
- How much weight have you gained?
- How often do you weigh yourself?

Retención de liquidos

¿Sufre Ud. de inflamación (hinchazón) del tobillo?

¿Le cuesta respirar por la noche?

¿Qué mejora los síntomas?

¿Qué empeora los síntomas?

¿Ha notado Ud. algún aumento de peso recientemente?
- ¿Cuánto peso ha aumentado?
- ¿Con cuánta frecuencia se pesa?

Shortness of breath

Do you have shortness of breath?
- How often?
- What makes it better?
- What makes it worse?

Do your lips or nail beds ever turn blue?
- When?

Does the position of your body affect your breathing?
- How?

Does time of day affect your breathing?
- What time of day do you have the most trouble breathing?

Does a particular activity affect your breathing?
- Bathing?
- Walking?
- Running?
- Climbing stairs?
- Other?

How many stairs can you climb before you feel short of breath?

Falta de aliento

¿Sufre Ud. de falta de aliento?
- ¿Con cuánta frecuencia?
- ¿Qué la mejora?
- ¿Qué la empeora?

¿Alguna vez los labios o el lecho de la uña se amoratan?
- ¿Cuándo?

¿La postura del cuerpo afecta su respiración?
- ¿Cómo?

¿Su respiración se ve afectada por el memento del día?
- ¿En qué momento del día tiene mayores dificultades para respirar?

¿Alguna actividad en particular afecta su respiración?
- ¿Bañarse?
- ¿Caminar?
- ¿Correr?
- ¿Subir escaleras?
- ¿Otra?

¿Cuántos escalones puede Ud. subir antes de que le falte el aliento?

How many blocks can you walk before you feel short of breath?

¿Cuántas cuadras puede caminar antes de que le falte el aliento?

What makes your breathing better?

¿Qué mejora su respiración?

Medical history

Have you had any lung problems?
– What type of problem?
– How long did it last?
– How was the problem treated?

¿Ha tenido Ud. problemas de los pulmones?
– ¿Qué tipo de problema?
– ¿Cuánto tiempo duró?
– ¿Qué tratamiento recibió?

Have you been exposed to anyone with a respiratory disease?

– What type of disease?
– When were you exposed to it?

¿Ha estado Ud. expuesto(a) a alguna persona que tenga una enfermedad respiratoria?
– ¿Qué clase de enfermedad?
– ¿Cuándo estuvo Ud. expuesto(a)?

Have you had chest surgery or any kind of test to diagnose a problem in your lungs?

– What type?
– Why did you have it?

¿Ha tenido Ud. cirugía de los pulmones o se le ha hecho un estudio diagnóstico de los pulmones?
– ¿Qué tipo?
– ¿Por qué tuvo la cirugía o por qué se le hizo el estudio?

When did you have your last chest X-ray?
– What was the result?

¿Cuándo se le tomó la última radiografía de los pulmones?
– ¿Qué indicaron los resultados?

When did you have your last tuberculosis test?
– What was the result?

¿Cuándo se le hizo el último análisis para la tuberculosis?
– ¿Qué indicaron los resultados?

In the last 1 to 2 months, have you had:
– fever?
– chills?
– fatigue?
– night sweats?

En los últimos dos meses ¿ha tenido:
– fiebre?
– escalofríos?
– fatiga?
– sudor nocturno?

Do you use any home remedies to help you breathe?
– What do you use?

¿Usa Ud. remedios caseros para sus problemas respiratorios?
– ¿Qué usa Ud.?

Do you have allergies that flare up in different seasons?

– What causes them?

¿Tiene Ud. alergias que se exacerban durante diferentes temporadas del año?
– ¿Qué es lo que las causa?

– Do your allergies cause:

    Runny nose?
    Itching eyes?

    Stuffy nose?
    Other symptoms?
– What do you do to relieve these symptoms?

Have you ever been vaccinated against flu or pneumonia?
– What type of vaccination did you receive?
– When did you receive it?

Have you ever had a blood test that showed you had anemia?

– When?

Do you ever have sinus pain?

– When?
– How is it treated?

Do you ever have nasal discharge or postnasal drip?
– When?
– How is it treated?

Do you ever have a bad taste in your mouth or have bad breath?
– When?

– ¿Le causan alguno de los siguientes síntomas?
    ¿Le gotea la nariz?
    ¿Tiene Ud. comezón en los ojos?
    ¿Se le congestiona la nariz?
    ¿Otros síntomas?
– ¿Qué hace Ud. para aliviar estos síntomas?

¿Se ha vacunado Ud. contra la gripe o pulmonía?
– ¿Qué tipo de vacuna se le administró?
– ¿Cuándo se vacunó?

¿Se le ha hecho un análisis de sangre que haya indicado que tenía anemia?
– ¿Cuándo?

¿Alguna vez le duelen los senos nasales?
– ¿Cuándo?
– ¿Qué tratamiento recibe?

¿Alguna vez ha tenido secreción nasal o goteo postnasal?
– ¿Cuándo?
– ¿Qué tratamiento recibe?

¿Alguna vez tiene Ud. mal sabor en la boca o mal aliento?

– ¿Cuándo?

Family history

Has any member of your family had:

– emphysema?
– asthma?
– respiratory allergies?

– tuberculosis?
    Did you have contact with the family member who had tuberculosis?
    When?

¿Algún miembro de su familia tuvo alguno de las siguientes enfermedades?
– ¿Enfisema?
– ¿Asma?
– ¿Alergias del sistema respiratorio?
– ¿Tuberculosis?
    ¿Estuvo Ud. en contacto con el miembro de la familia que tuvo tuberculosis?
    ¿Cuándo?

Health patterns

<table>
<tr><td>

Medications

Do you use a nebulizer or other breathing treatment?
– What condition does it treat?

– What dose do you use?
– How often do you give yourself a treatment?
– Do you ever experience side effects from the treatment?

– Do you follow special instructions for giving yourself the treatment?
– When did you last give yourself a treatment?

Do you use oxygen at home?
– Do you use a cannula or a mask?
– How often do you use it?
– What is the flow rate of oxygen?

    At rest?
    With activity?
– Do you use an oxygen concentrator?
– Do you use portable oxygen?

– Must you follow special instructions?
– How long have you been using oxygen at home?

Do you take medications?
– Prescription?
– Over-the-counter?
– Home remedies
– Herbal preparations
– Other?

Which prescription medications do you take?
– How often do you take them?

Which over-the-counter medications do you take?
– How often do you take them?

</td><td>

Medicamentos

¿Usa Ud. un nebulizador u otro tratamiento para respirar?
– ¿Para qué condición usa Ud. el tratamiento?
– ¿Qué dosis se le dió?
– ¿Con qué frecuencia administra Ud. un tratamiento?
– ¿Alguna vez tiene Ud. efectos secundarios a causa del tratamiento?
– ¿Sigue Ud. instrucciones especiales para el uso del tratamiento?
– ¿Cuándo se realizó el último tratamiento?

¿Usa Ud. oxígeno en casa?
– ¿Usa Ud. una cánula o máscara?

– ¿Con qué frecuencia la usa?
– ¿Cuál es la tasa de flujo de un litro de oxígeno?
    ¿En reposo?
    ¿En actividad?
– ¿Usa un concentrador de oxigeno?
– ¿Usa oxígeno portátil?

– ¿Tiene Ud. que seguir instrucciones especiales?
– ¿Hace cuánto tiempo que Ud. usa oxígeno en casa?

¿Toma Ud. medicamentos?
– ¿Con receta?
– ¿De venta libre?
– ¿Remedios caseros?
– ¿Preparados herbales?
– ¿Otro?

¿Qué medicamentos de receta toma Ud.?
– ¿Con qué frecuencia los toma?

¿Qué medicamentos de venta libre toma?
– ¿Con qué frecuencia los toma?

</td></tr>
</table>

Why do you take these medications?

¿Por qué toma Ud. estos medicamentos?

How much of each medication do you take?

¿Qué dosis toma Ud. de cada uno de estos medicamentos?

How does each medication make you feel?

¿Cómo le hace sentirse cada uno de estos medicamentos?

Are you allergic to any medication?
- Which medications?
- What happens when you have an allergic reaction?

¿Es Ud. alérgico(a) a algún medicamento?
- ¿Qué medicamentos?
- ¿Qué pasa cuando Ud. tiene una reacción alérgica?

Personal habits

Hábitos personales

Do you smoke or chew tobacco?

¿Fuma Ud. o masca tabaco?

- What do you smoke?
  Cigarettes?
  Cigars?
  Pipe?
- How long have you smoked or chewed tobacco?
- How many cigarettes, cigars, or pipes of tobacco do you smoke each day?
- How much tobacco do you chew each day?
- Did you ever stop?

  For how long?
  What method did you use to stop?
  What made you decide to stop?
- Do you remember why you started again?

- ¿Qué fuma Ud.?
  ¿Cigarrillos?
  ¿Cigarros (puros)?
  ¿Pipa?
- ¿Hace cuánto tiempo que Ud. fuma o masca tabaco?
- ¿Cuántos cigarrillos, cigarros (puros) o pipas de tabaco fuma Ud. al día?
- ¿Cuánto tabaco masca Ud. a diario?
- ¿Dejó Ud. alguna vez de fumar o mascar tabaco?
  ¿Cuánto tiempo duró?
  ¿Qué método usó Ud. para dejar de fumar o mascar?
  ¿Qué hizo que decidiera dejar de fumar?
- ¿Recuerda Ud. por qué volvió a comenzar a fumar o mascar tabaco otra vez?

If you do not use tobacco now, have you smoked or chewed tobacco in the past?

Si Ud. no usa tabaco actualmente, ¿ha Ud. fumado o mascado tabaco en el pasado?

Do you drink alcoholic beverages?
- What type?
  Beer?
  Wine?
  Hard liquor?
- How often do you drink alcoholic beverages?

¿Bebe Ud. bebidas alcohólicas?
- ¿Qué clase?
  ¿Cerveza?
  ¿Vino?
  ¿Aguardiente?
- ¿Con qué frecuencia bebe bebidas alcohólicas?

– How many drinks do you have in one day?
> Spread over how much time?

– ¿Cuántos tragos toma en un día?
> ¿Repartidas en cuánto tiempo?

Sleep patterns

How many hours do you sleep each night?

When you wake up, do you feel rested?

Do you snore?

How many pillows do you use when sleeping?
– Are you using more or fewer pillows than you used to?

Have your breathing problems changed the way you sleep?

Have you ever been told that you have sleep apnea?
– When?
– What treatment are you receiving for sleep apnea?

Patrones de sueño

¿Cuántas horas duerme por noche?

Cuando se despierta, ¿se siente bien descansado?

¿Ronca?

¿Cuántas almohadas usa Ud. para dormir?
– ¿Usa Ud. más o menos almohadas que las que usaba antes?

¿Ha cambiado su manera de dormir a causa de sus problemas de respiración?

¿Ya le han dicho que tiene apnea de sueño?
> ¿Cuándo?
> ¿Qué tratamiento ésta recibiendo para la apena del sueño?

Activities

Does your breathing problem affect your daily activities?

– How?

How do your current activities compare with those before your breathing problems started?

Do you play sports?
– Which sports?
– How often?
– Do they affect your breathing?
> How?

Do you have any hobbies that expose you to glues, paints, sprays, or other irritants that could cause breathing problems?

Actividades

¿Su problema de respiración afecta sus actividades cotidianas?
– ¿Cómo?

¿Cómo se comparan sus actividades actuales con las anteriores a sus problemas del sistema respiratorio?

¿Practica deportes
– ¿Qué deportes?
– ¿Con qué frecuencia?
– ¿Afectan su respiración?
> ¿Cómo?

¿Tiene pasatiempos favoritos que lo (la) exponen a pegamentos, pinturas, rociadores u otros agentes irritantes del sistema respiratorio?

Nutrition

Do you have any trouble breathing when you are eating?
– What happens?

Describe what you usually eat each day.

Are you on a special diet?
– What kind of diet?

Have you gained weight recently?
– How much?

Have you lost weight recently?

– How much?

Sexual patterns

Has your breathing problem affected your sex life?

– How?

Environment

Do you live in a house or in an apartment?
– Are there steps in your home?
– On which level are the bedroom, bathroom, and kitchen?

Does anyone in your home smoke?

How many people live with you?

Do you have pets?
– Does your pet's fur or feathers bother you?
– How does it bother you?
  Runny nose?
  Cough?
  Other?

How is your home heated?

Is there anything in your home that could cause breathing problems?
– Fresh paint?

Nutrición

¿Tiene Ud. dificultad para respirar cuando come?
– ¿Qué ocurre?

Describa lo que generalmente come cada día.

¿Tiene una dieta especial?
– ¿Qué tipo de dieta?

¿Ha aumentado de peso recientemente?
– ¿Cuánto?

¿Ha bajado de peso recientemente?
– ¿Cuánto?

Patrones sexuales

¿Su problema respiratorio ha afectado su actividad sexual de algún modo?
– ¿Cómo?

Entorno

¿Vive en casa o departamento?

– ¿Hay escalones en su casa?
– ¿En qué piso están la habitación, el baño y la cocina?

¿Fuma alguien en su casa?

¿Cuántas personas viven con Ud.?

¿Tiene Ud. animales?
– ¿Le molestan a Ud. el pelaje o las plumas del animal?
– ¿Cómo le molestan?
  ¿Le gotea a Ud. la nariz?
  ¿Tose?
  ¿Otro?

¿Qué tipo de calefacción tiene Ud. en casa?

¿Hay algo en su casa que le pueda provocar problemas respiratorios?
– ¿Pintura fresca?

– Cleaning sprays?
– Cigarette smoke?
– Other?

– ¿Rociadores de limpieza?
– ¿Humo de cigarrillo?
– ¿Otro?

Do you have air conditioning?

¿Tiene aire acondicionado?

Do you have a dehumidifier?

¿Tiene un deshumidificador?

Do certain weather conditions affect your symptoms?

¿Hay determinadas condiciones climáticas que afecten sus síntomas?

– What are they?
– How do they affect you?

– ¿Cuáles?
– ¿Cómo lo afectan?

Are you exposed to any known respiratory irritants at work?

¿En su trabajo está Ud. expuesto(a) a agentes irritantes que le afecten la respiración, que Ud. sepa?

– Do you use safety measures when you are exposed to them?

– ¿Usa Ud. medidas de seguridad mientras está expuesto(a)?

Psychosocial considerations

Coping skills

Habilidad de sobrellevar problemas

Does stress at home or work affect the way you breathe?

¿El estrés en casa o en el trabajo le afecta la respiración?

Do you do anything special to manage your stress?
– What do you do?

¿Aplica Ud. algunas medidas especiales para tratar el estrés?
– ¿Cuáles son?

Roles

Roles

How has your breathing problem affected you and your family?

¿Qué impacto ha tenido su enfermedad respiratoria en Ud. y en su familia?

How have family members reacted to your breathing problem?

¿Cómo han reaccionado los miembros de la familia a su enfermedad respiratoria?

Do you have family and friends you can depend on for support?

¿Tiene familia o amistades de quienes Ud. puede depender para que le den apoyo?

Responsibilities

Responsabilidades

What is your current occupation?

¿Cuál es su ocupación de trabajo actual?

What were your previous occupations?

¿Cuáles fueron sus ocupaciones de trabajo anteriores?

Can you afford the medications, equipment, and oxygen you need to manage your breathing problem?	¿Puede Ud. afrontar el gasto de medicamentos, el equipo y el oxígeno necesario para su enfermedad respiratoria?
Do you have health insurance?	¿Posee cobertura de salud?
Are you able to meet your family responsibilities?	¿Puede cumplir con las responsabilidades de familia?

Developmental considerations

For the pediatric patient

Para el (la) paciente de pediatría

Did the mother have any pregnancy-related problems?	¿Tuvo la madre problemas relacionados con el embarazo?
Did she carry the pregnancy to term? – What care did the premature infant require?	¿Llegó el embarazo a su término? – ¿Qué cuidado necesitó el (la) infante(a) prematuro(a)?
Did the infant have any breathing problems at birth? – How were they treated?	¿Tuvo el (la) infante(a) problemas respiratorios al nacer? – ¿Qué tratamiento se les dió?
Does the infant have frequent congestion, runny nose, or colds?	¿Sufre el (la) infante(a) de frecuente congestión, goteo de nariz o catarro?
Does shortness of breath interfere with the infant's ability to nurse?	¿La falta de aliento interfiere con la habilidad de mamar del (de la) infante(a)?
Does the child cough at night? – Does the cough waken the child?	¿Tose el (la) niño(a) por la noche? – ¿Se despierta el (la) niño(a) cuando tose?
Does coughing or shortness of breath interfere with the child's play or school activities?	¿La tos o la falta de aliento interfiere con el juego o con las actividades escolares del niño (de la niña)?

For the pregnant patient

Para la paciente embarazada

Have you had any breathing problems during your pregnancy? – What kind? – How often? – What makes them better? – What makes them worse?	¿Tuvo algún problema respiratorio durante su embarazo? – ¿De qué tipo? – ¿Con cuánta frecuencia? – ¿Qué lo mejora? – ¿Qué lo empeora?

For the elderly patient	Para el (la) paciente anciano(a)
Are you aware of any changes in the way you breathe?	¿Es Ud. consciente de algún cambio en su manera de respirar?
Do you tire easily when you are climbing stairs?	¿Se fatiga Ud. con facilidad al subir escaleras?
Do you have trouble breathing when you are lying flat?	¿Tiene Ud. dificultad en respirar cuando se acuesta de espaldas?
Do you seem to have more colds? – Do they last longer?	¿Le parece que se resfría con mayor frecuencia? – ¿Duran más los resfríos?

12

Cardiovascular system

Current health problems

Chest pain

Do you ever have chest pain or discomfort?
– How would you characterize the pain or discomfort?
 Constant?
 Intermittent?

Where in your chest do you feel the pain?
– Point to where you feel the pain.

Does the pain go to any other area?

Does your chest hurt more when you touch it?

What does the pain feel like?
– Crushing or squeezing?
– Someone or something heavy is pressing on your chest?
– Tightness?
– Dull ache?
– Burning?
– Sharp or stabbing, like a knife?

– Ripping or tearing?

How long have you been having this chest pain?
– Did it start in the past few hours, days, or weeks?
– Did it start suddenly or slowly?

How long does the pain last?

– Seconds?
– Minutes?

Dolor de pecho

¿Alguna vez siente dolor o molestia en el pecho?
– ¿Cómo lo describiría?

 ¿Constante?
 ¿Intermitente?

¿En qué parte del pecho siente Ud. el dolor?
– ¿Puede Ud. señalar con el dedo dónde siente el dolor?

¿Se extiende este dolor a otra parte del cuerpo?

¿Le duele más el pecho cuando lo toca?

¿Qué clase de dolor es?
– ¿Agobiante?
– ¿Cómo si alguien o algo pesado estuviera oprimiendo su pecho?
– ¿Tensión?
– ¿Dolor sordo?
– ¿Ardor?
– ¿Agudo o punzante, como un cuchillo?
– ¿Sensación desgarrante?

¿Hace cuánto tiempo que Ud. tiene este dolor de pecho?
– ¿Hace unas horas, días o semanas?
– ¿Comenzó súbita o lentamente?

¿Cuánto tiempo dura un acceso?
– ¿Segundos?
– ¿Minutos?

Heart
El corazón

Pulmonary valve
La válvula pulmonar

Superior vena cava
La vena cava superior

Branches of right pulmonary artery
Las ramas de la arteria pulmonar derecha

Branches of right pulmonary vein
Las ramas de la vena pulmonar derecha

Right atrium
El atrio derecho

Chordae tendineae
La cuerda tendinosa

Tricuspid valve
La válvula tricúspide

Right ventricle
El ventrículo de la derecha

Inferior vena cava
La vena cava inferior

Papillary muscle
El músculo papilar

Descending aorta
La aorta descendiente

Aortic arch
El arco de la aorta

Pulmonary trunk
El tronco pulmonar

Branches of left pulmonary artery
Las ramas de la arteria pulmonar izquierda

Branches of left pulmonary vein
Las ramas de la vena pulmonar izquierda

Left ventricle
Ventrículo lizquierdo

Myocardium
El miocardio

Left atrium
El atrio izquierdo

Mitral valve
Válvula mitral

Aortic valve
Válvula de la aorta

Interventricular septum
Septum interventricular

– Hours?
– Days?

What makes the pain better?

– ¿Horas?
– ¿Días?

Qué alivia el dolor?

Coronary circulation
La circulación coronaria

Anterior view
Vista anterior

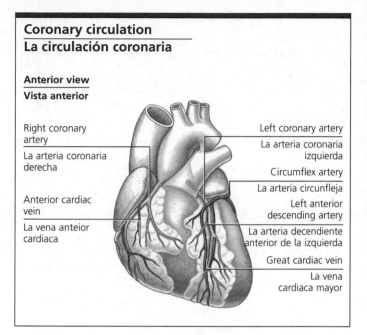

Right coronary artery
La arteria coronaria derecha

Anterior cardiac vein
La vena anteior cardiaca

Left coronary artery
La arteria coronaria izquierda

Circumflex artery
La arteria circunfleja

Left anterior descending artery
La arteria decendiente anterior de la izquierda

Great cardiac vein
La vena cardiaca mayor

What makes the pain worse?

What other symptoms do you have with the pain?
– Trouble breathing?
– Sweating?
– Nausea?

¿Qué empeora el dolor?

¿Qué otros sínotomas acompañan el dolor?
– ¿Dificultad para respirar?
– ¿Sudoración?
– ¿Náuseas?

Dizziness

Do you ever feel dizzy or light-headed when you change positions?
– When do you feel this way?
    Changing from lying to sitting?
    Changing from sitting to standing?
    Other?

Mareo

¿Hay veces cuando Ud. se marea al cambiar de postura?

– ¿Cuándo ocurre?
    ¿Cuando se sienta después de estar acostado(a)?
    ¿Cuando se para después de estar sentado(a)?
    ¿En otra ocasión?

Fatigue

Do you tire more easily than you used to?

What type of activity makes you feel tired?

Fatiga

¿Se cansa Ud. con más facilidad que antes?

¿Qué tipo de actividad le hace sentirse cansado?

What makes you feel less tired?	**¿Qué lo hace sentir menos cansado?**
What makes you feel more tired?	**¿Qué lo hace sentir más cansado?**

Fluid retention | Retención de líquidos

Do your shoes or rings feel tight?	**¿Le aprietan los zapatos o los anillos?**
Do your ankles or feet swell?	**¿Siente Ud. que se le hinchan los tobillos o los pies?**
– When does this happen?	– ¿Cuándo?
– What makes it better?	– ¿Qué lo alivia?
– What makes it worse?	– ¿Qué lo empeora?

Palpitations | Palpitaciones

Does your heart ever feel like it is pounding, racing, or skipping beats?	**¿Siente Ud. alguna vez que el corazón le golpea, le late aceleradamente o se entrecortan los latidos?**
– How often does this happen?	– ¿Con qué frecuencia?
– What does it feel like?	– ¿Cómo se siente cuando esto ocurre?
– Do you feel faint when this happens?	– ¿Siente mareos cuando esto ocurre?
When does this feeling happen?	**¿Cuándo ocurre esta sensación?**
– While resting?	– ¿Al descansar?
– During an activity?	– ¿Al hacer alguna actividad?
– After an activity, such as exercising or walking up steps?	– ¿Después de una actividad, tal como hacer ejercicio o subir escalones?
– After eating?	– ¿Después de comer?
What makes the feeling better?	**¿Qué alivia la sensación?**
What makes the feeling worse?	**¿Qué intensifica la sensación?**

Shortness of breath | Falta de aliento

Have you ever had trouble catching your breath?	**¿Alguna vez ha sentido Ud. que le falta el aliento?**
– When did it occur?	– ¿Cuándo ocurrió?
– Does it happen often?	– ¿Ocurre a menudo?
Is it related to any activity?	**¿Está relacionada con alguna actividad?**
– Which activity?	– ¿Con qué actividad?
Is it accompanied by coughing?	**¿Va acompañada de tos?**
What makes it better?	**¿Qué la alivia?**

What makes it worse?	**¿Qué la empeora?**

Skin ulcerations

Do you have any ulcers or sores on your legs?
– Are they getting better or worse?

How long have you had them?

Have you ever had them treated?

How were they treated?

Do you notice any change in how your legs or feet feel?

Ulceración de la piel

¿Tiene Ud. úlceras o llagas en las piernas?
– ¿Se están mejorando o empeorando?

¿Hace cuánto tiempo que las tiene?

¿Alguna vez ha recibido Ud. tratamiento por ellas?

¿Qué tratamiento se les dió?

¿Ha notado Ud. algún cambio en la sensación en las piernas o los pies?

Medical history

Were you born with a heart condition?
– When was it treated?
– How was it treated?

Have you had rheumatic fever?

– When?

Do you have any heart problems because of the rheumatic fever?

Have you ever been told you had a heart murmur?
– Who told you about it?
– When did you find out about it?

Do you have:
– high blood pressure?
– high cholesterol?
– diabetes mellitus?

– other conditions?
    When was the disorder first diagnosed?

    How do you manage it?

¿Nació Ud. con algún problema cardiaco?
– ¿Cuándo recibió tratamiento?
– ¿Cómo se le trató?

¿Ha tenido Ud. fiebre reumática?
– ¿Cuándo?

¿Ha tenido enfermedades del corazón como consecuencia de la fiebre reumática?

¿Alguna vez se le ha dicho que tenía un soplo cardiaco?
– ¿Quién se lo dijo?
– ¿Cuándo se enteró Ud. de esto?

¿Tiene Ud.:
– presión sanguínea alta?
– colesterol alto?
– diabetes melitus (trastorno metabólico caracterizado por la disminución o pérdida de la capacidad para oxidar los carbohidratos)?
– otras afecciones?
    ¿Cuándo se le diagnosticó por primera vez este trastorno?
    ¿Cómo lo controla?

How has it affected your lifestyle?

¿Cómo le ha afectado su modo de vida?

Have you experienced:
– chest pain?
– arm or jaw pain?

– shortness of breath?
– fainting or dizziness?
– foot or ankle swelling?
– rapid heartbeats?
– bluish discoloration of your skin?

When did this happen?
How long did it last?

¿Ha tenido Ud.:
– dolor de pecho?
– dolor en los brazos o la mandíbula?
– falta de respiración?
– desmayo o mareo?
– hinchazón de pie o tobillo?
– palpitaciones?
– decoloración azulada de la piel?

¿Cuándo ocurrió esto?
¿Cuánto tiempo duró?

Have you ever been confused?

– When?
– For how long did it last?

¿Se ha sentido Ud. desorientado?

– ¿Cuándo?
– ¿Por cuánto tiempo?

Have you felt unusually tired in the past few months?
– What made you feel so tired?
– How frequently do you feel like this?

¿Ha sentido un cansancio inusual en los últimos meses?
– ¿Cuál fue la causa?
– ¿Con qué frecuencia se ha sentido así?

Have you had dental work or an invasive procedure, such as cystoscopy or endoscopy, within the past few weeks?

– Which procedure did you have?
– When was it done?

En las últimas semanas, ¿se le ha hecho un trabajo dental o ha tenido un procedimiento invasivo, como una cistoscopia o endoscopia?
– ¿Qué procedimiento fue?
– ¿Cuándo se lo realizaron?

Have you ever had an allergic reaction to a medication?

– Which medication?
– How would you describe the reaction?

¿Ha tenido Ud. alguna vez una reacción alérgica a algún medicamento?
– ¿A qué medicamento?
– ¿Cómo describiría Ud. la reacción?

Have you ever had an electrocardiogram?
– What were the results?

¿Alguna vez le hicieron un electrocardiograma?
– ¿Cuáles fueron los resultados obtenidos?

When did you last have a chest X-ray?

– What were the results?

¿Cuándo fue la última vez que le realizaron una ecografía del pecho?
– ¿Cuáles fueron los resultados obtenidos?

Family history

Has anyone in your family been treated for heart disease?

– How is that person related to you?
– What kind of heart disease did the person have?
– At what age did the disease develop?

Has anyone in your family died suddenly of an unknown cause?
– Who?
– At what age?

Does anyone in your family have high blood pressure, high cholesterol, or diabetes mellitus?
– At what age did the disease develop?
– How is it treated?

¿Algún miembro de su familia ha recibido tratamiento por alguna enfermedad cardiaca?

– ¿Cómo está Ud. emparentado con esa persona?
– ¿Qué trastorno tuvo?

– ¿A qué edad le ocurrió?

¿Algún miembro de su familia ha muerto repentinamente por causa desconocida?
– ¿Quién?
– ¿A qué edad?

¿Hay alguien en su familia que tenga la presión sanguínea alta, colesterol alto, o diabetes melitus?
– ¿A qué edad se le desarrolló la enfermedad?
– ¿Qué tratamiento recibe?

Health patterns

Medications

Do you take any medications?
– Prescription?
– Over-the-counter?
– Home remedies?
– Herbal preparations?
– Other?

Which prescription medications do you take?
– How often do you take them?

Which over-the-counter medications do you take?
– How often do you take them?

Why do you take these medications?

How much of each medication do you take?

Medicamentos

¿Toma Ud. medicamentos?
– ¿Con receta?
– ¿De venta libre?
– ¿Remedios caseros?
– ¿Preparados herbales?
– ¿Otros?

¿Qué medicamentos con receta toma Ud.?
– ¿Con qué frecuencia los toma?

¿Qué medicinas de venta libre toma Ud.?
– ¿Con qué frecuencia las toma?

¿Por qué toma Ud. estos medicamentos?

¿Qué dosis toma de cada medicamento?

How does each medication make you feel?

Are you allergic to any medications?
- Which medications?
- What happens when you have an allergic reaction?

Personal habits

Do you smoke or chew tobacco?
- What do you smoke?
    Cigarettes?
    Cigars?
    Pipe?
- How long have you smoked or chewed tobacco?
- How many cigarettes, cigars, or pipes of tobacco do you smoke per day?
- How much tobacco do you chew per day?
- Did you ever stop smoking?
    For how long?

    What made you decide to stop?
    What method did you use to stop?
- Do you remember why you started again?

If you do not use tobacco now, have you smoked or chewed tobacco in the past?

Do you drink alcoholic beverages?
- What type?
    Beer?
    Wine?
    Hard liquor?
- How often do you drink alcoholic beverages?
- How many drinks do you have in one day?
    Spread over how much time?

¿Cómo le hace sentirse cada uno de estos medicamentos?

¿Es Ud. alérgico(a) a algún medicamento?
- ¿A qué medicamentos?
- ¿Qué pasa cuando Ud. tiene una reacción alérgica?

Hábitos personales

¿Fuma Ud. o masca tabaco?
- ¿Qué fuma?
    ¿Cigarrillos?
    ¿Cigarros (puros)?
    ¿Pipa?
- ¿Hace cuánto tiempo que fuma o masca tabaco?
- ¿Cuántos cigarrillos, cigarros (puros) o pipas de tabaco fuma Ud. al día?
- ¿Cuánto tabaco masca al día?
- ¿Dejó Ud. el hábito alguna vez?
    ¿Cuánto tiempo duró sin fumar?
    ¿Qué hizo que decidiera dejar de fumar?
    ¿Qué método usó Ud. para dejar de fumar?
- ¿Recuerda Ud. por qué volvió a fumar o mascar tabaco?

Si no consume tabaco actualmente, ¿ha fumado o mascado tabaco en el pasado?

¿Toma Ud. bebidas alcohólicas?
- ¿Qué clase?
    ¿Cerveza?
    ¿Vino?
    ¿Aguardiente?
- ¿Con qué frecuencia toma bebidas alcohólicas?
- ¿Cuántos tragos toma en un día??
    ¿Repartidas en cuánto tiempo?

Sleep patterns	Patrones de sueño

How many hours do you sleep each night?

¿Cuántas horas duerme Ud. cada noche?

When you wake up, do you feel rested?

¿Se siente Ud. descansado a la mañana siguiente?

Do you feel tired later in the day?

¿Se siente Ud. cansado más tarde en el día?

Do you take naps?
- When do you take them?
- How long do you nap?

¿Toma Ud. siestas?
- ¿Cuándo las toma?
- ¿Por cuánto tiempo duerme la siesta?

Have you been told that you snore?

¿Se le ha dicho que ronca?

Do you wake up during the night to urinate?

¿Se despierta Ud. durante la noche para orinar?

Do you cough or have short-ness of breath during the night?
- When?
- How frequently?
  Every night?
  A few times per week?

  A few times per month?

¿Tiene Ud. accesos de falta de aliento o tos durante la noche?

- ¿Cuándo?
- ¿Con qué frecuencia ocurren?
  ¿Todas las noches?
  ¿Unas cuantas veces a la semana?
  ¿Unas cuantas veces al mes?

Do you become short of breath when you lie flat?

¿Le falta el aliento cuando se acuesta de espaldas?

How many pillows do you use at night?
- Has this number changed re-cently?
- Do the pillows help you breathe?

¿Cuántas almohadas usa Ud. en la noche?
- ¿Ha cambiado últimamente este número?
- Las almohadas, ¿lo ayudan a respirar?

Activities	Actividades

How would you describe your typical day?

¿Cómo describiría un día típi-co?

Do you exercise regularly?

¿Hace Ud. ejercicio rutinaria-mente?

- Which exercises do you do?
- How often do you exercise?

- How hard do you exercise?

- How much time do you spend exercising?

- ¿Qué tipo de ejercicio hace?
- ¿Con qué frecuencia hace ejerci-cio?
- ¿Con qué intensidad hace el ejercicio?
- ¿Por cuánto tiempo hace Ud. ejercicio?

Did a health care professional prescribe your exercise plan?

– Who?

Do environmental factors, such as very hot or cold temperatures, humidity, or pollution, affect your ability to exercise?

– Do any of these factors affect the way you feel after exercise?

Has your exercise level changed from what it was six months, one year, or five years ago?
– How has it changed?

Have you noticed any change in your ability to do the things you do every day (such as dressing, grooming, walking, or eating)?

Do you have any hobbies or play any sports?
– How frequently do you engage in them?
– How do you feel after these activities?
– Has your level of involvement in these activities changed recently?
– What caused this change?

When you walk or exercise, do you have leg pain?

Nutrition

What have you eaten during the past three days?

Do you follow a special diet?

– What kind of diet?
– Did a health care professional prescribe this diet for you?

Do you eat at fast-food restaurants?

¿Una persona especialista en el cuidado de la salud le recetó su plan de ejercicios?
– ¿Quién fue?

¿Las circunstancias ambientales, como temperaturas extremas, la humedad o la contaminación, afectan su capacidad de hacer ejercicio?
– ¿Cualquiera de esos factores le afecta la manera de sentirse después de hacer ejercicio?

¿Ha cambiado su nivel de ejercicio con respecto a hace seis meses, un año o cinco años?

– ¿De qué manera cambió?

¿Ha notado Ud. algún cambio en su capacidad de realizar las actividades normales de su vida cotidiana (tal como vestirse, asearse, caminar o comer)?

¿Tiene algún pasatiempo o practica algún deporte?
– ¿Con qué frecuencia se dedica a él?
– ¿Cómo se siente Ud. después de participar en estas actividades?
– ¿Ha cambiado recientemente su grado de participación en estas actividades?
– ¿Qué fue lo que causó este cambio?

Cuando camina o hace ejercicio, ¿tiene Ud. dolor de piernas?

Nutrición

¿Qué ha comido Ud. en los últimos tres días?

¿Sigue Ud. alguna dieta especial?
– ¿Qué clase de dieta?
– Esta dieta, ¿se la recetó una persona especialista en el cuidado de la salud?

¿Come Ud. en restaurantes de comida rápida?

– How often?
– What do you usually order?

– ¿Con qué frecuencia?
– ¿Por lo general, qué platos pide?

Does your ethnic or cultural background affect the way you eat?
– How?

¿Su origen étnico o cultural ejerce una influencia sobre su dieta?
– ¿Cómo?

Does your religion affect what you eat?

– How?

¿Su religión limita, o de cualquier modo afecta, lo que Ud. come?
– ¿Cómo lo afecta?

Have you gained any weight recently?
– If so, how much?

¿Ha aumentado de peso últimamente?
– Si ha aumentado, ¿cuánto?

Have you lost any weight recently?
– If so, how much?

¿Ha bajado Ud. de peso últimamente?
– Si ha bajado, ¿cuánto?

Sexual patterns

Has your sex life changed in any way?

Patrones sexuales

¿Ha cambiado, en cualquier forma, su actividad sexual?

Environment

Do you live in a house or in an apartment?
– How many floors does your home have?
– Must you climb steps to get inside?
– Must you climb steps to get from room to room?
– How many?
– On which level are the bathroom, bedroom, and kitchen located?

Entorno

¿Vive Ud. en una casa o en un apartamento?
– ¿Cuántos pisos tiene?

– ¿Tiene Ud. que subir escalones para entrar?
– ¿Tiene que subir escalones para ir de un cuarto a otro?
– ¿Cuántos?
– ¿En qué piso están el baño, la recámara y la cocina?

Do certain weather conditions make your symptoms better or worse?
– What are these conditions?
– How do they affect your symptoms?

¿Las condiciones climáticas afectan sus síntomas?

– ¿Cuáles son estas condiciones?
– ¿Qué efecto tienen en sus síntomas?

Psychosocial considerations

Coping skills

What makes you stressed?
- How often does this happen?
- What physical feelings do you have when you are stressed?

Do you feel pressured to complete tasks in a short time?

Do you rush from one job or task to another?

How do you cope with the stress in your life?

Habilidad de sobrellevar problemas

¿Qué le hace sentirse estresado?
- ¿Con qué frecuencia siente esto?
- ¿Qué síntomas físicos tiene Ud. cuando está estresado?

¿Se siente presionado a terminar una tarea en poco tiempo?

¿Se apura para ir de un trabajo o tarea a otro?

¿Cómo maneja el estrés en su vida?

Roles

Do you think of yourself as a healthy person or sick person?
- What makes you feel this way?
- Do you feel that your health problem has changed your life?

Roles

¿Se considera Ud. una persona saludable o enfermiza?
- ¿Qué le hace sentirse así?
- ¿Cree Ud. que su problema de salud ha cambiado su vida?

Responsibilities

What are your typical responsibilities at home?

What are the typical responsibilities of your spouse and children?

Have your responsibilities at home changed since you developed a health problem?
- How do you feel about these changes?

Do you have a job?
- What is your occupation?
- How many hours per day do you work?
- How many days per week do you work?
- What are your responsibilities at work?
- What are the physical demands of the job?
- How much lifting do you do?

Responsabilidades

¿Cuáles son sus responsabilidades típicas en casa?

¿Cuáles son las responsabilidades típicas de su cónyuge y de sus hijos?

¿Han cambiado sus responsabilidades en casa desde que tuvo un problema de salud?
- ¿Qué siente acerca de estos cambios?

¿Tiene trabajo?
- ¿Cuál es su profesión o trabajo?
- ¿Cuántas horas a la semana trabaja Ud.?
- ¿Cuántos días por semana?

- ¿Cuáles son sus responsabilidades?
- ¿Cuáles son las exigencias físicas de su trabajo?
- ¿Cuántos objetos debe levantar Ud.?

– How much walking do you do?

– ¿Cuánto tiene Ud. que caminar?

– Do you work outside?

– ¿Trabaja al aire libre?

– Is the place where you work:
  hot?
  cold?
  humid?
  dusty?
  smoky?
  noisy?

– El lugar donde trabaja:
  ¿es caluroso?
  ¿es frío?
  ¿es húmedo?
  ¿es polvoriento?
  ¿está lleno de humo?
  ¿es ruidoso?

Do your financial resources and insurance cover your medical needs and preventive measures?

¿Sus recursos financieros y seguro cubren sus necesidades medicinales y medidas preventivas?

Developmental considerations

For the pediatric patient

Para el (la) paciente de pediatría

Has the child experienced any growth delay?

¿Ha tenido el (la) niño(a) un retraso en su desarrollo?

Does the child have any problems with coordination?

¿Tiene el (la) niño(a) algún problema de coordinación?

Does the child turn blue when he or she cries?

¿Se pone amoratado el (la) niño(a) cuando llora?

During play, does the child stop frequently to sit or squat?

¿Deja de jugar el (la) niño(a) con frecuencia para sentarse o acuclillarse?

Does the child have trouble eating?

¿Tiene el (la) niño(a) dificultad en alimentarse?

Does the child tire easily or sleep a lot?

¿Se cansa con facilidad el (la) niño(a) o duerme demasiado?

Does the child frequently develop strep throat or a sore throat and fever?

¿Tiene el (la) niño(a) con frecuencia inflamación de garganta o dolor de garganta?

For the pregnant patient

Para la paciente embarazada

During this pregnancy, has any health care professional told you that you have a heart murmur?

¿Durante este embarazo, le ha dicho algún profesional de la salud que tiene un soplo cardiaco?

Do you ever feel dizzy or lightheaded when you change positions or exert yourself?

¿Se siente Ud. mareada después de cambiar de postura o de hacer un trabajo pesado?

Has your blood pressure been elevated during this pregnancy?

¿Ha subido su presión sanguínea durante este embarazo?

Have you noticed any swelling in your feet or ankles?

¿Ha notado Ud. alguna hinchazón de los pies o de los tobillos?

Have you developed varicose veins in your legs or genitals?

¿Se le han formado venas varicosas en las piernas o los genitales?

Have you developed hemorrhoids?

¿Se le han formado hemorroides?

Does your heart pound after stress or exertion?

¿Le late el corazón violentamente después de una gran tensión o fatiga?

Do you suffer from shortness of breath?
– Do you cough or wheeze when you have shortness of breath?

¿Se queda Ud. sin aliento?
– Esta falta de aliento, ¿va acompañada de tos o de respiración jadeante?

For the elderly patient

Para el (la) paciente aciano(a)

Do you feel cold even when the temperature is warm?

¿Siente frio aun cuando la temperatura es cálida?

Do you have more episodes of chest pain than when you were younger?

¿Tiene más episodios de dolor de pecho que cuando era más joven?

13

Gastrointestinal system

Current health problems

Changes in bowel habits

Cambio de los hábitos de evacuación intestinal

When did you last have a bowel movement or pass gas?

¿Cuándo fue la última vez que Ud. tuvo una evacuación intestinal o gases?

How often do you have regular bowel movements?

¿Con qué frecuencia tiene Ud. evacuaciones intestinales regulares?

– Once daily?
– More than once daily?
– Every other day?
– Other?

– ¿Una vez al día?
– ¿Más de una vez al día?
– ¿Un día sí y un día no?
– ¿Otra?

What color are your stools?

¿De qué color es su materia decal?

– Brown?
– Black?
– Red?
– Clay-colored?
– Green?
– Other?

– ¿Café?
– ¿Negro?
– ¿Rojo?
– ¿Color de arcilla?
– ¿Verde?
– ¿Otro?

Have you noticed any change in your normal pattern of bowel movements?
– How has it changed?
    Stools more frequent?
    Stools less frequent?

¿Ha notado Ud. algún cambio en el patrón regular de sus evacuaciones intestinales?
– ¿Cómo ha cambiado?
    ¿Defeca con más frecuencia?
    ¿Defeca con menos frecuencia?

Are the stools formed or loose?

¿Su materia fecal es sólida o líquida?

– Are formed stools soft or hard?

– ¿Su materia fecal sólida es blanda o dura?

– Are the stools liquid?

– Su materia fecal, ¿es líquida?

Do you have difficulty passing stools?

¿Tiene dificultad para defecar?

Gastrointestinal system
El sistema gastrointestinal

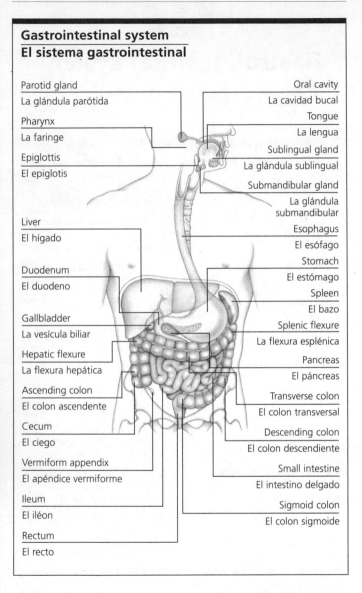

Parotid gland
La glándula parótida

Pharynx
La faringe

Epiglottis
El epiglotis

Liver
El hígado

Duodenum
El duodeno

Gallbladder
La vesícula biliar

Hepatic flexure
La flexura hepática

Ascending colon
El colon ascendente

Cecum
El ciego

Vermiform appendix
El apéndice vermiforme

Ileum
El iléon

Rectum
El recto

Oral cavity
La cavidad bucal

Tongue
La lengua

Sublingual gland
La glándula sublingual

Submandibular gland
La glándula submandibular

Esophagus
El esófago

Stomach
El estómago

Spleen
El bazo

Splenic flexure
La flexura esplénica

Pancreas
El páncreas

Transverse colon
El colon transversal

Descending colon
El colon descendiente

Small intestine
El intestino delgado

Sigmoid colon
El colon sigmoide

Do you suffer from constipation?

– When did it start?

– How often are you constipated?

¿Sufre Ud. de estreñimiento?

– ¿Cuándo comenzó a sufrir de esto?

– ¿Con cuánta frecuencia se constipa?

Do you have any pain when you are constipated?
- Where is the pain?
- How often do you have the pain?
- How long does it last?
- What makes it better?
- What makes it worse?

Have you noticed swelling in your abdomen?

Do you have other symptoms, such as cramping?

¿Tiene dolor cuando se constipa?
- ¿Dónde se localiza el dolor?
- ¿Con qué frecuencia siente el dolor?
- ¿Cuánto dura?
- ¿Qué lo alivia?
- ¿Qué lo intensifica?

¿Ha notado inflamación del abdomen?

¿Tiene Ud. otros síntomas, tal como retortijones?

Difficulty swallowing

Do you have any difficulty swallowing?
- When did this problem start?
- When does it occur?
    With all foods?
    With liquids?

Do you cough after you swallow?

Dificultad para tragar

¿Tiene Ud. dificultad para tragar?
- ¿Cuándo comenzó el problema?
- ¿Cuándo ocurre esto?
    ¿Con todos los alimentos?
    ¿Con los líquidos?

¿Tose depués de tragar?

Indigestion

Do you have heartburn or indigestion?
- When does it occur?
    Morning?
    Afternoon?
    Evening?
    During sleep?

Is this problem associated with eating?
- How long does the feeling last?
- What did you eat?

What makes the problem better?

What makes the problem worse?

Indigestión

¿Sufre de acidez estomacal o indigestión?
- ¿Cuándo la tiene?
    ¿Por la mañana?
    ¿Por la tarde?
    ¿Por la noche?
    ¿Mientras Ud. duerme?

¿Se relaciona esta indigestión con la comida?
- ¿Cuánto dura la sensación?
- ¿Qué comió Ud.?

¿Qué mejora el problema?

¿Qué empeora el problema?

Loss of appetite

Have you had a recent change in appetite?
- What kind of change?

Have you had a recent change in diet?

Pérdida de apetito

¿Ha tenido Ud. recientemente un cambio en su apetito?
- ¿Qué clase de cambio?

¿Ha tenido Ud. recientemente un cambio de dieta?

– What kind of change?

– ¿Qué clase de cambio?

Do any specific foods or liquids bother you?

¿Hay algunos alimentos o líquidos en particular que le molestan?

– Which foods or liquids?

– ¿Qué alimentos o qué líquidos?

Nausea and vomiting

Náuseas y vómitos

Have you had any nausea?

¿Ha tenido Ud. náuseas?

– When does it occur?

– ¿Cuándo las tiene?

– How often does it occur?

– ¿Con qué frecuencia?

Did you vomit?

¿Vomitó Ud.?

– How much did you vomit?

– ¿Cuánto vomitó?

– What color was the vomitus?

– ¿De qué color fue el vómito?

– How many times did you vomit?

– ¿Cuántas veces vomitó?

Did you notice any blood in the vomitus?

¿Notó Ud. algo de sangre en lo que vomitó?

– How much blood was present?

– ¿Cuánta sangre había?

Did the vomitus have a fecal odor?

¿Lo que Ud. vomitó tenía un olor fecal?

Pain

Dolor

Do you have any pain?

¿Tiene Ud. algún dolor?

– Point to where you have the pain.

– Señale el lugar donde siente el dolor.

What does the pain feel like?

¿Qué tipo de dolor siente Ud.?

– Burning?

– ¿Ardiente?

– Squeezing?

– ¿Siente que se retuerce?

– Dull?

– ¿Sordo?

– Sharp or stabbing?

– ¿Agudo o punzante?

– Being tied in knots?

– ¿Siente nudos?

Does the pain make it hard for you to walk?

¿Le molesta el dolor cuando camina?

– Can you walk upright while you have the pain?

– ¿Puede Ud. caminar derecho(a)?

Were you drinking alcohol before the stomach pain began?

¿Estaba Ud. tomando bebidas alcohólicas antes que le comenzara el dolor de estómago?

– How much alcohol did you drink?

– ¿Cuánto alcohol bebió?

– What type?

– ¿De qué tipo?

What makes the pain better?

¿Qué alivia el dolor?

What makes the pain worse?

¿Qué intensifica el dolor?

When does the pain occur?
- Before meals?
- Immediately after meals?

- Two to three hours after meals?

Do you have other signs or symptoms when you have this pain?
- Fever?
- Weak or sick feeling?
- Nausea?
- Diarrhea?
- Vomiting?
- Swelling, such as in the mouth?

¿Cuándo siente Ud. el dolor?
- ¿Antes de las comidas?
- ¿Inmediatamente después de las comidas?
- ¿Dos o tres horas después de las comidas?

¿Tiene Ud. otros síntomas junto con el dolor?

- ¿Fiebre?
- ¿Debilidad?
- ¿Náuseas?
- ¿Diarrea?
- ¿Vómito?
- ¿Hinchazón, por ejemplo en la boca?

Weight loss

How much do you weigh?

Have you recently lost weight without trying?

- How much weight did you lose?
- Over how long a period of time?

Pérdida de peso

¿Cuánto pesa?

¿Ha tenido Ud. recientemente una pérdida de peso no intencional?
- ¿Cuánto peso ha bajado?
- ¿Durante cuánto tiempo?

Medical history

Have you had any major illnesses, trauma, extensive dental work, hospitalizations, or chronic medical conditions?

- What were they?
- When did they occur?
- How were they treated?

Have you ever had an eating disorder, such as anorexia nervosa or bulimia?

Have you had problems with your mouth, throat, abdomen, or rectum that have lasted for a long time?
- When did the problem occur?

- How long did it last?
- How was it treated?

¿Ha tenido Ud. alguna enfermedad grave, trauma, extenso trabajo dental, hospitalizaciones o algunas condiciones médicas crónicas?
- ¿Cuáles?
- ¿Cuándo se produjeron?
- ¿Cómo se trataron?

¿Ha sufrido Ud. de algún trastorno relacionado con la comida, tal como anorexia nerviosa o bulimia?

¿Ha tenido Ud. algún problema con la boca, la garganta, el abdomen o el recto que haya durado por mucho tiempo?
- ¿Cuándo se produjo el problema?
- ¿Cuánto duró?
- ¿Cómo fue tratado?

Have you ever had surgery on your mouth, throat, abdomen, or rectum?

¿Ha tenido Ud. alguna vez cirugía de la boca, la garganta, el abdomen o el recto?

Are you allergic to milk products or other foods?

¿Tiene Ud. alguna alergia a alimentos, tal como los productos lácteos?

– What happens when you have an allergic reaction?

– ¿Qué pasa cuando Ud. tiene una reacción alérgica?

Do you have trouble breathing?

¿Tiene Ud. dificultad para respirar?

Have you lived in or traveled to a foreign country?
– When?
– Where?

¿Ha vivido Ud. o viajado por algún país en el extranjero?
– ¿Cuándo?
– ¿Dónde?

Have you noticed any swelling in your neck, underarms, or groin?
– When did it start?

¿Ha notado Ud. alguna hinchazón en el cuello, las axilas o la ingle?
– ¿Cuándo comenzó?

Have you had any nerve problems, such as weakness or numbness in your hands and fingers?
– When did it start?
– How long did it last?
– How was it treated?

¿Ha tenido Ud. algún problema con los nervios, tal como debilidad o adormecimiento en las manos o los dedos?
– ¿Cuándo comenzó?
– ¿Cuánto duró?
– ¿Cómo fue tratado?

Do you have eye pain, tearing, redness, or intolerance to light?

– When does it occur?

¿Le duelen o lagrimean los ojos o están enrojecidos o no toleran la luz?
– ¿Cuándo?

Family history

Does anyone in your family have a history of:
– Heart disease?
– Crohn's disease?
– Diabetes mellitus?
– Gastrointestinal tract disorders?

– Sickle cell anemia?
– Food intolerance?
– Obesity?

¿Hay algún miembro de su familia que tenga un historial de:
– enfermedad cardiovascular?
– enfermedad de Crohn?
– diabetes mellitus?
– afecciones en la región gastrointestinal?
– drepanocitosis?
– intolerancia a alimentos?
– obesidad?

Has anyone in your family had colon or rectal cancer or polyps?
– Who?

¿Hay algún miembro de su familia que haya tenido cáncer del recto o del colon o pólipos?
– ¿Quién?

- When was it diagnosed?
- How was it treated?

Has anyone in your family had colitis?
- Who?
- When was it diagnosed?
- How was it treated?

– ¿Cuándo se le diagnosticó?
– ¿Qué tratamiento se le dió?

¡Hay algún miembro de su familia que haya tenido colitis?
– ¿Quién?
– ¿Cuándo se le diagnosticó?
– ¿Qué tratamiento se le dió?

Health patterns

Medications

Do you take any medications?
- Prescription?
- Over-the-counter?
- Home remedies?
- Herbal preparations?
- Other?

Which prescription medications do you take?
- How often do you take them?

Which over-the-counter medications do you take?
- How often do you take them?

Why do you take these medications?

How much of each medication do you take?

How does each medication make you feel?

Are you allergic to any medications?
- Which medications?
- What happens when you have an allergic reaction?

Do you use laxatives?
- How often?

Do you use enemas?
- How often?

Do you take:

- Vitamin supplements?
- Mineral supplements?
- Appetite suppressants?

Medicamentos

¡Toma Ud. medicamentos?
– ¿Con receta?
– ¿De venta libre?
– ¡Remedios caseros?
– ¿Preparados herbales?
– ¿Otro?

¡Qué medicamentos de receta toma Ud.?
– ¿Con qué frecuencia los toma?

¡Qué medicamentos de venta libre toma?
– ¿Con qué frecuencia los toma?

¿Por qué toma Ud. estos medicamentos?

¿Cuál es la dosis para cada uno de estos medicamentos?

¿Cómo le hace a Ud. sentirse cada uno de estos medicamentos?

¡Es Ud. alérgico(a) a algunos medicamentos?
– ¿Qué medicamentos?
– ¿Qué le pasa cuando tiene una reacción alérgica?

¡Usa laxantes?
– ¿Con qué frecuencia?

¡Usa Ud. enemas?
– ¿Con qué frecuencia?

¡Toma Ud. alguno de los siguientes?
– ¿Suplemento de vitaminas?
– ¿Suplemento de minerales?
– ¿Supresores del apetito?

Who prescribed them?

¿Quién se los recetó?

Why do you take them?

¿Por qué los toma Ud.?

When did you start taking them?

¿Cuándo comenzó Ud. a tomarlos?

How much of them do you take?

¿Qué cantidad toma?

How frequently do you take them?

¿Con qué frecuencia los toma?

| Personal habits | Hábitos personales |

Do you smoke or chew tobacco?

¿Fuma Ud. o masca tabaco?

– What do you smoke?
　　Cigarettes?
　　Cigars?
　　Pipe?
– How long have you smoked or chewed tobacco?
– How many cigarettes, cigars, or pipes of tobacco do you smoke per day?
– How much tobacco do you chew per day?
– Did you ever stop?

　　For how long?

　　What made you decide to stop?
　　What method did you use to stop?
　　Do you remember why you started again?

– ¿Qué fuma Ud.?
　　¿Cigarrillos?
　　¿Cigarros (puros)?
　　¿Pipa?
– ¿Hace cuánto tiempo que Ud. fuma o masca tabaco?
– ¿Cuántos cigarrillos, cigarros (puros) o pipas de tabaco fuma al día?
– ¿Cuánto tabaco masca Ud. al día?
– ¿Dejó Ud. de fumar o mascar tabaco alguna vez?
　　¿Cuánto tiempo duró sin fumar o mascar tabaco?
　　¿Qué hizo que decidiera dejar de fumar?
　　¿Qué método usó Ud. para dejar el hábito?
　　¿Recuerda Ud. por qué comenzó otra vez?

If you do not use tobacco now, have you in the past?

Si Ud. no consume tabaco actualmente, ¿ha fumado o mascado tabaco en el pasado?

Do you drink alcoholic beverages?

¿Toma Ud. bebidas alcohólicas?

– What type?
　　Beer?
　　Wine?
　　Hard liquor?
– How often do you drink alcoholic beverages?
– How many drinks do you have in one day?
　　Spread over how much time?

– ¿Qué clase?
　　¿Cerveza?
　　¿Vino?
　　¿Aguardiente?
– ¿Con qué frecuencia toma bebidas alcohólicas?
– ¿Cuántos tragos toma en un día?
　　¿Distribuidos a lo largo de cuánto tiempo?

Sleep patterns

How many hours do you sleep each night?

When you wake up, do you feel rested?

Do gastrointestinal symptoms ever wake you at night?
- What happens?
- What relieves the symptoms?

- What do you do to get back to sleep?

Activities

What do you do during the day?
- How do these activities make you feel?
- Does your gastrointestinal problem interfere wih these activities?
    How?

Do you exercise?
- What kind of exercise do you do?
- Why do you exercise?

    Pleasure?
    Conditioning?
    Control your weight?
    Build muscle?
- How often do you exercise?

    For how long?

Do you have trouble moving or feel pain in your joints?

- When does it occur?

Nutrition

What foods do you eat during the day?

Are you on a special diet?
- What type of diet?

Patrones de sueño

¿Cuántas horas duerme por noche?

Cuando se despierta, ¿se siente bien descansado?

Los sítomas gastointestinales, ¿lo despiertan de noche?
- ¿Qué pasa?
- ¿Qué es lo que le mitiga los síntomas?
- ¿Qué hace Ud. para volver a dormirse?

Actividades

¿Qué tipo de actividades hace Ud. de día?
- ¿Cómo le hacen sentir estas actividades?
- Sus problemas gastrointestinales, ¿interfieren con estas actividades?
    ¿Cómo?

¿Hace Ud. ejercicio?
- ¿Qué clase de ejercicio hace Ud.?
- ¿Cuáles son las razones por las que Ud. hace ejercicio?
    ¿Por placer?
    ¿Para ponerse en forma?
    ¿Para controlar el peso?
    ¿Para la estructura muscular?
- ¿Con qué frecuencia hace Ud. ejercicio?
    ¿Durante cuánto tiempo?

¿Tiene Ud. alguna dificultad con los movimientos del cuerpo o dolor en las articulaciones?
- ¿Cuándo occure?

Nutrición

¿Qué come Ud. durante el transcurso de un día?

¿Tiene una dieta especial?
- ¿Qué tipo de dieta?

Are there foods you believe you should not eat?
– What are these foods?
– Why do you believe that you should not eat these foods?
– How do these foods affect you?

¿Hay alimentos que Ud. sabe que no debería comer?
– ¿Cuáles son estos?
– ¿Por qué cree Ud. que no debiera comerlos?
– ¿Cómo le afectan estos alimentos que Ud. come?

How many servings do you drink of _____ each day?
– coffee
– tea
– cola
– cocoa
– water

¿Cuántas porciones ingiere al día de _____?
– café
– té
– bebidas cola
– chocolate
– agua

How do you care for your teeth and gums?
– Do tooth or gum problems make it hard for you to eat?

¿Qué cuidado le da Ud. a los dientes y las encías?
– ¿Tiene Ud. algún problema con los dientes o las encías que interfieran con su capacidad de comer?

Who does the food shopping for your household?

¿Quién hace sus compras de comestibles?

Do you have adequate storage and refrigeration?

¿Tiene Ud. alacenas y un refrigerador adecuados?

Who prepares the meals?

¿Quién prepara las comidas?

Where is your food prepared?

¿Dónde se preparan los alimentos?

Do you eat alone or with others?

¿Come Ud. solo(a) o con otros?

Sexual patterns

Patrones sexuales

Do you have anal sex?

¿Practica el sexo anal?

Has your current problem affected your sex life?
– How?

Su problema actual, ¿ha afectado su vida sexual?
– ¿Cómo?

Environment

Entorno

Do you live in a house or in an apartment?
– How many floors does your home have?
– Where is the bathroom?

¿Vive Ud. en una casa o en un apartamento?
– ¿Cuántos pisos tiene?
– ¿Dónde está el baño?

Can you get to the bathroom to move your bowels?
– If not, what do you do when you need to move your bowels?

¿Puede Ud. llegar hasta el baño para evacuar?
– Si no puede llegar, ¿qué hace cuando necesita evacuar?

Psychosocial considerations

Coping skills

Have you recently lost a loved one, ended a relationship, or experienced a similarly stressful event?

Have you been depressed or anxious recently?

Does the stress of your job, daily schedule, or other factors influence your eating or bowel patterns?

– How?

Do you use food or drink to help you get through a stressful event?

Roles

Do you like the way you look?

Are you content with your present weight?

Responsibilities

What is your occupation?

How do you feel about your job?

Do you receive financial assistance for food?
– What type of assistance?
　　Food stamps?

　　Social Security payments?

　　Supplemental Social Security payments?
　　Welfare?
　　Women, infants, and children (WIC) program?

Habilidad de sobrellevar problemas

¿Últimamente se le ha muerto alguna persona querida, ha roto sus relaciones personales con una persona amada o ha sufrido algún acontecimiento lleno de tensiones similares?

¿Se ha sentido Ud. deprimido(a) o preocupado(a) últimamente?

¿Su tensión en el trabajo, su horario diario, u otros factores influyen en sus hábitos de comer o en su evacuación intestinal?
– ¿Cómo?

¿Toma Ud. alimentos o bebidas para que le ayuden a superar situaciones estresantes?

Roles

¿Le gusta su aspecto físico?

¿Está Ud. satisfecho(a) con su peso actual?

Responsabilidades

¿Cuál es su profesión o trabajo?

¿Qué opina Ud. de su trabajo?

¿Recibe Ud. alguna forma de asistencia para los alimentos?
– ¿Qué clase de asistencia?
　　¿Estampillas de asistencia para comprar alimentos?
　　¿Mensualidad del Seguro Social?
　　¿Complemento a la mensualidad del Seguro Social?
　　¿Asistencia social?
　　¿Programa de WIC (mujeres, infantes y niños)?

Developmental considerations

For the pediatric patient

Para el (la) paciente de pediatría

Is your infant breast-fed or bottle-fed?

Su criatura, ¿es amamantada o alimentada con biberón?

What is the color of the newborn's stools?

¿De qué color es la materia fecal del (de la) recién nacido(a)?

How many stools per day does the newborn pass each day?

¿Cuántas veces defeca el (la) recién nacido(a) al día?

Does your infant continually want to eat despite vomiting forcefully?

¿Quiere comer continuamente el (la) infante(a) a pesar de que vomita todo?

How often does the child have a bowel movement?

¿Con qué frecuencia evacua la criatura?

Are the child's stools soft, hard, or runny?

La materia fecal de la criatura es blanda, dura o líquida?

What color are the stools?

¿De qué color es la materia fecal?

What special words does the child use for having a bowel movement?

¿Cuáles son las palabras especiales que el (la) niño(a) usa para decir que quiere evacuar?

At what age was the child toilet-trained?
– Did the child have trouble learning to use the toilet?

¿A qué edad aprendió al (la) niño(a) a usar el retrete?
– ¿Tuvo problemas con esto?

Does the child seem to have more "accidents" when ill?

¿Tiene la criatura más "accidentes" cuando está enferma?

Are the child's underpants often stained with stool?

¿Los calzones del (de la) niño(a) están manchados de heces con frecuencia?

Do you suspect that the child sometimes deliberately holds back stool?

¿Sospecha Ud. que a veces la criatura intencionalmente retiene la defecación?

Do the child's stools ever appear large, bulky, and frothy? Do they float in the toilet bowl?

¿Hay veces que la materia fecal del (la) niño(a) parece ser grande, abultada y espumosa y flota en el retrete?

– Is the odor especially strong?

– ¿Es el olor especialmente fuerte?

Is the child under unusual stress?

¿Está la criatura bajo una tensión inusual?

For the pregnant patient

Do you ever experience nausea and vomiting?
- Do they occur at a specific time?
- Do they occur throughout the day?
- How long has the nausea and vomiting been happening?
- How much do you vomit?

Have your bowel habits changed since you became pregnant?
- How have they changed?

Have you had abdominal pain?

- Where is the pain?
- What kind of pain is it?
- When does the pain occur?
- How long does it last?
- What makes it better?
- What makes it worse?

Have you had heartburn?
- When does it occur?
- How long does it last?
- What makes it better?
- What makes it worse?

Have you had any problems with constipation?
- How often?
- What makes it better?
- What makes it worse?

For the elderly patient

Do you ever lose control of your bowels?

Are you constipated frequently?

- Does this represent a change in your normal bowel habits?

Para la paciente embarazada

¿Tiene Ud. alguna vez náuseas o vómitos?
- ¿Ocurre esto a una hora en particular?
- ¿Ocurre esto durante todo el día?
- ¿Cuánto hace que tiene náuseas y vómitos?
- ¿Cuánto vomita?

¿Han cambiado sus hábitos de defecación desde el comienzo de su embarazo?
- ¿Cómo han cambiado?

¿Ha tenido Ud. dolor en el abdomen?
- ¿Dónde es el dolor?
- ¿Qué clase de dolor?
- ¿Cuándo se produce el dolor?
- ¿Cuánto dura?
- ¿Qué lo alivia?
- ¿Qué lo intensifica?

¿Ha tenido acidez estomacal?
- ¿Cuándo se produce?
- ¿Cuánto dura?
- ¿Qué lo alivia?
- ¿Qué lo intensifica?

¿Ha tenido algún problema de constipación?
- ¿Con cuánta frecuencia?
- ¿Qué lo alivia?
- ¿Qué lo empeora?

Para el (la) paciente anciano(a)

¿Hay veces en que no controla sus intestinos?

¿Está Ud. estreñido(a) con frecuencia?
- ¿Representa esto un cambio en sus hábitos normales de defecación?

Do you have diarrhea after eating certain foods?

– What foods seem to cause diarrhea?

Do you need help to use the bathroom?

¿Le da diarrea después de comer ciertos alimentos?

– ¿Qué alimentos parecen darle diarrea?

¿Necesita Ud. ayuda para ir al baño?

14

Urologic system

Current health problems

Changes in urinary elimination patterns

How often do you urinate each day?
- How much urine do you pass each time?

How does your bladder feel after you urinate?
- Full?
- Empty?

What color is your urine?
- Light yellow?
- Dark yellow?
- Red?
- Brown?
- Black?

Does your urine ever appear cloudy?
- How often does this occur?

Burning

Do you ever feel a burning sensation when you urinate?
- How often?

Where do you feel the burning sensation?
- At the urethral opening?
- Around the area of the urethral opening?
- Inside the urethra?

Cambios en los patrones de evacuación urinaria

¿Con qué frecuencia orina Ud. al día?
- ¿Cuánta orina elimina cada vez?

¿Cómo se siente su vejiga después de orinar?
- ¿Llena?
- ¿Vacía?

¿De qué color es su orina?
- ¿Amarilla pálida?
- ¿Amarilla oscura?
- ¿Roja?
- ¿Café?
- ¿Negra?

¿Hay veces que la orina parece estar turbia?
- ¿Con qué frecuencia ocurre esto?

Sensación de ardor

¿Hay veces que Ud. siente ardor cuando orina?
- ¿Con qué frecuencia?

¿Dónde siente Ud. el ardor?

- ¿En la abertura de la uretra?
- ¿Alrededor de la abertura de la uretra?
- ¿Dentro de la uretra?

Kidney
El riñón

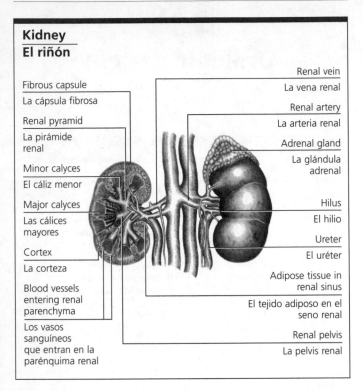

Fibrous capsule
La cápsula fibrosa

Renal pyramid
La pirámide renal

Minor calyces
El cáliz menor

Major calyces
Las cálices mayores

Cortex
La corteza

Blood vessels entering renal parenchyma
Los vasos sanguíneos que entran en la parénquima renal

Renal vein
La vena renal

Renal artery
La arteria renal

Adrenal gland
La glándula adrenal

Hilus
El hilio

Ureter
El uréter

Adipose tissue in renal sinus
El tejido adiposo en el seno renal

Renal pelvis
La pelvis renal

Hesitancy	Vacilación
Do you ever have trouble starting or maintaining a urine stream?	**¿Hay veces que Ud. tiene dificultad en comenzar a orinar o mantener un flujo de orina?**
– How often does this occur?	– ¿Con qué frecuencia ocurre esto?
Have you noticed a change in the size or force of your urine stream?	**¿Ha notado Ud. algún cambio en el tamaño o la fuerza del flujo de su orina?**
– Can you describe it?	– ¿Lo puede Ud. describir?

Pain	Dolor
Do you ever have pain when you urinate?	**¿Alguna vez siente Ud. dolor al orinar?**
– How often?	– ¿Con qué frecuencia?
Every time?	¿Todas las veces?
Frequently?	¿Con frecuencia?
Occasionally?	¿De vez en cuando?
Where is the pain located?	**¿Dónde siente Ud. el dolor?**
– At the urethral opening?	– ¿En la abertura de la uretra?

– Around the area of the urethral opening?

– Inside the urethra?

– In the lower abdomen?

– In the lower back?

What does the pain feel like?
– Burning?
– Squeezing?
– Dull or aching?
– Sharp or stabbing?
– Heaviness?
– Spasms?

What makes the pain better?

What makes the pain worse?

Do you ever have pain in your back, below your ribs?

Urethral discharge

Do you ever have urethral discharge?
– How much discharge have you noticed?
– What color is the discharge?
– Does the discharge have any odor?
   What kind of odor?

How long have you had this discharge?

Has the amount of the discharge increased or decreased?

Urgency

Do you ever feel that you must urinate immediately?

– How often do you have this feeling?

Do you ever feel this way, then are not able to urinate?

Urine leakage

Do you ever leak urine?

– ¿Alrededor de la abertura de la uretra?

– ¿Dentro de la uretra?

– ¿En la parte inferior del abdomen?

– ¿En la parte inferior de la espalda?

¿Qué tipo de dolor siente Ud.?
– ¿Una sensación de ardor?
– ¿Siente que se retuerce?
– ¿Sordo o doliente?
– ¿Agudo o punzante?
– ¿Una sensación de pesadez?
– ¿Espasmos?

¿Qué alivia el dolor?

¿Qué intensifica el dolor?

¿Alguna vez tiene Ud. dolor por debajo de las costillas cerca de la espalda?

Secreción de la uretra

¿Hay veces que Ud. tiene una descarga de la uretra?
– ¿Cuánta secreción ha notado Ud.?
– ¿De qué color es la secreción?
– ¿Tiene olor la secreción?

   ¿Qué clase de olor?

¿Hace cuánto tiempo que tiene Ud. esta secreción?

¿Ha aumentado o disminuido la cantidad de esta secreción?

Urgencia

¿Hay veces que Ud. siente que tiene que orinar inmediatamente?
– ¿Con qué frecuencia ocurre esto?

¿Alguna vez se siente así y luego no puede orinar?

Pérdida de orina

¿Tiene Ud. pérdida de orina?

– When does it occur?
    When you laugh, sneeze, or
      cough?
    During exercise?
    When you bend to pick
      something up?
    When you change positions?

    When you strain to move
      your bowels?
    After you feel the urge to
      urinate?
– How often does it occur?

**How long have you had this
leakage?**

**Do you wear absorbent pads to
prevent soiling your clothes?**

– ¿Cuándo la tiene?
    ¿Cuándo Ud. se ríe, estornu-
      da o toce?
    ¿Cuándo Ud. hace ejercicio?
    ¿Cuándo se agacha Ud. a
      recoger algo?
    ¿Cuándo Ud. cambia de pos-
      tura?
    ¿Cuándo se esfuerza Ud.
      para evacuar?
    ¿Después de sentir urgencia
      de orinar?
– ¿Con qué frecuencia ocurre esto?

**¿Hace cuánto tiempo que Ud.
tiene esta pérdida de orina?**

**¿Usa Ud. una toalla higiénica
para evitar manchar su ropa?**

Medical history

**Have you ever had a kidney or
bladder problem, such as a urinary tract infection?**

– What was the problem?
– When did it first occur?

– How was it treated?

**Have you ever had kidney or
bladder stones?**
– When?
– How were they treated?

**Have you ever had a kidney or
bladder injury?**
– What kind of injury?
– When did the injury occur?
– How was it treated?

**Have you ever had a catheter
put into your bladder or another part of your body?**
– Why?
– Did you have any problems
  while you were using the
  catheter?

**Have you ever had a sexually
transmitted disease?**

**¿Ha tenido Ud. alguna vez un
problema del riñón o de la vejiga, tal como una infección en el
sistema urinario?**
– ¿Cuál fue el problema?
– ¿Cuándo ocurrió por primera
  vez?
– ¿Qué tratamiento se le dió?

**¿Ha tenido Ud. alguna vez cál-
culos en el riñón o en la vejiga?**
– ¿Cuándo?
– ¿Qué tratamiento se le dió?

**¿Ha tenido Ud. alguna vez una
lesión del riñón o de la vejiga?**
– ¿Qué tipo de lesión?
– ¿Cuándo la tuvo?
– ¿Qué tratamiento se le dió?

**¿Alguna vez le han insertado
un catéter en la vejiga u otra
parte del cuerpo?**
– ¿Por qué?
– ¿Tuvo Ud. problemas mientras
  tenía colocado el catéter?

**¿Ha tenido Ud. alguna vez algu-
na enfermedad de transmisión
sexual?**

– Which disease did you have?
    Chlamydia?
    Gonorrhea?
    Syphilis?
    Another sexually transmitted disease?
– How long ago did you have this disease?
– How was it treated?

Are you being treated for a medical problem, such as diabetes mellitus or high blood pressure?
– What is the problem?
– When did it start?
– How is it treated?

– ¿Qué enfermedad?
    ¿Clamidia?
    ¿Gonorrea?
    ¿Sífilis?
    ¿Otra enfermedad de transmisión sexual?
– ¿Hace cuánto tiempo la tuvo?

– ¿Qué tratamiento se le dió?

¿Actualmente recibe Ud. un tratamiento para un problema médico, tal como diabetes mellitus o alta presión sanguínea?
– ¿Cuál es el problema?
– ¿Cuándo comenzó?
– ¿Cómo se lo trata?

Family history

Has anyone in your family ever been treated for kidney problems?
– Who?
– What kind of problem was it?
– How was it treated?

Has anyone in your family ever had kidney or bladder stones?

– Who?
– When?
– How was the problem treated?

Has anyone in your family ever had:
– high blood pressure?
– diabetes mellitus?
– gout?
– coronary artery disease?

    Who?
    How was it treated?

¿Hay algún miembro de su familia tratado a causa de un problema del riñón?
– ¿Quién es?
– ¿Qué clase de problema?
– ¿Qué tratamiento se le dió?

¿Hay algún miembro de su familia que haya tenido cálculos en el riñón o en la vejiga?

– ¿Quién?
– ¿Cuándo?
– ¿Qué tratamiento se le dió?

¿Hay algún miembro de su familia que haya tenido:
– alta presión sanguínea?
– diabetes mellitus?
– gota?
– enfermedad de la arteria coronaria?

    ¿Quién?
    ¿Qué tratamiento se le dió?

Health patterns

Medications

Do you take any medications?
– Prescription?
– Over-the-counter?

Medicamentos

¿Toma Ud. medicamentos?
– ¿Con receta?
– ¿De venta libre?

– Home remedies?
– Herbal preparations?
– Other?

Which prescription medications do you take?
– How often do you take them?

Which over-the-counter medications do you take?
– How often do you take them?

Why do you take these medications?

How much of each medication do you take?

How does each medication make you feel?

Are you allergic to any medications?
– Which medications?
– What happens when you have an allergic reaction?

Personal habits

Do you smoke or chew tobacco?
– What do you smoke?
    Cigarettes?
    Cigars?
    Pipe?
– How long have you smoked or chewed tobacco?
– How many cigarettes, cigars, or pipes of tobacco do you smoke each day?
– How much tobacco do you chew each day?
– Did you ever stop?

    For how long?
    What made you decide to stop?
    What method did you use to stop?
    Do you remember why you started again?

– ¿Remedios caseros?
– ¿Preparados herbales?
– ¿Otro?

¿Qué medicamentos de receta toma Ud.?
– ¿Con qué frecuencia los toma?

¿Qué medicamentos de venta libre toma?
– ¿Con qué frecuencia los toma?

¿Por qué toma Ud. estos medicamentos?

¿Qué dosis toma de cada medicamento?

¿Cómo le hace sentirse cada medicamento?

¿Está Ud. alérgico(a) a algunos medicamentos?
– ¿A qué medicamentos?
– ¿Qué pasa cuando Ud. tiene una reacción alérgica?

Hábitos personales

¿Fuma Ud. o masca tabaco?

– ¿Qué fuma Ud.?
    ¿Cigarrillos?
    ¿Cigarros (puros)?
    ¿Pipa?
– ¿Hace cuánto tiempo que Ud. fuma o masca tabaco?
– ¿Cuántos cigarrillos, cigarros (puros) o pipas de tabaco fuma Ud. al día?
– ¿Cuánto tabaco masca Ud. al día?
– ¿Dejó Ud. de fumar o mascar tabaco alguna vez?
    ¿Cuánto tiempo duró?
    ¿Qué lo hizo decidirse a dejar de fumar?
    ¿Qué método usó Ud. para dejar el hábito?
    ¿Recuerda Ud. por qué volvió a fumar o mascar tabaco otra vez?

If you do not use tobacco now, have you smoked or chewed tobacco in the past?

Si Ud. no consume tabaco actualmente, ¿ha Ud. fumado o mascado tabaco en el pasado?

Do you drink alcoholic beverages?
- What type?
  Beer?
  Wine?
  Hard liquor?
- How often do you drink alcoholic beverages?
- How many drinks do you have in one day?
  Spread over how much time?

¿Toma Ud. bebidas alcohólicas?
- ¿Qué clase?
  ¿Cerveza?
  ¿Vino?
  ¿Aguardiente?
- ¿Con qué frecuencia toma bebidas alcohólicas?
- ¿Cuántos tragos toma en un día?
  ¿Repartidas en cuánto tiempo?

Sleep patterns

Patrones de sueño

How many hours do you sleep each night?

¿Cuántas horas duerme por noche?

When you wake up, do you feel rested?

Cuando se despierta, ¿se siente bien descansado?

Do you have to get up at night to urinate?
- How often does this happen?

- How long has this been happening?

¿Se levanta de noche a orinar?

- ¿Con qué frecuencia ocurre esto?
- ¿Hace cuánto tiempo que le pasa esto?

Does this happen only when you drink a lot of liquid in the evening?

¿Le pasa esto solamente cuando ha bebido grandes cantidades de líquido en la noche?

Do you ever notice that your pajamas or sheets are soiled with urine?

¿Ha notado Ud. alguna vez que sus pijamas o las sábanas están manchadas de orina?

Nutrition

Nutrición

Do you follow a special diet?
- What kind of diet?
- Who prescribed the diet?
- How long have you been on the diet?
- Why do you follow the diet?

¿Tiene Ud. una dieta especial?
- ¿Qué clase de dieta?
- ¿Quién le recetó la dieta?
- ¿Hace cuánto tiempo que tiene Ud. esta dieta?
- ¿Cuál es la razón por la cual Ud. tiene esta dieta?

Do you limit the amount of salt you use?
- Why?
- How much salt do you use?

¿Limita Ud. la cantidad de sal que ingiere?
- ¿Por qué?
- ¿Cuánta sal usa?

How many glasses of liquid do you drink each day?

¿Cuántos vasos de líquido toma Ud. al día?

What type of liquid do you drink?

¿Qué tipo de líquidos bebe Ud.?

Sexual patterns

Patrones sexuales

Do you ever have pain during sex?

¿Hay veces que Ud. siente dolor cuando tiene relaciones sexuales?

Has your current problem affected your sex life?
– How?

Su problema actual, ¿ha afectado su vida sexual?
– ¿Cómo?

Environment

Entorno

Do you live in a house or in an apartment?
– How many floors does your home have?
– Where is the bathroom?

¿Vive Ud. en una casa o en un apartamento?
– ¿Cuántos pisos tiene?

– ¿Dónde está el baño?

Can you get to the bathroom when you have to urinate?
– If not, what do you do when you have to urinate?

¿Puede Ud. llegar hasta el baño cuando tiene que orinar?
– Si no puede llegar, ¿qué hace cuando tiene que orinar?

Psychosocial considerations

Roles

Roles

Can you urinate without help?
– If you need help, what kind of help do you need?

¿Puede Ud. orinar sin ayuda?
– ¿Qué clase de ayuda necesita Ud.?

If you have to urinate frequently or have to urinate at night, does this affect any family members?
– How?

¿Si Ud. tiene que orinar con frecuencia o tiene que orinar durante la noche, esto afecta a algún miembro de la familia?
– ¿Cómo?

Responsibilities

Responsabilidades

What is your occupation?

¿Cuál es su profesión o su trabajo?

Do you have enough time to visit the bathroom while you work?

¿Tiene tiempo suficiente para ir al baño mientras Ud. está en su trabajo?

Developmental considerations

For the pediatric patient

Does the child have a diaper rash that will not go away?

– When does it occur?
– What, if anything, relieves the rash?

How many diapers does the child wet each day?
– Has this number changed recently?
    Decreased?
    Increased?

Is the child thirsty often?

How much liquid does the child drink each day?
– What kinds of liquid?

Has the child experienced recent urinary problems?
– How would you describe the problem?

Does the child cry when urinating?

Has the child's bladder control deteriorated recently?

Did the child learn to sit, stand, and talk at the expected time?

Does the child have a schedule for urinating, such as always urinating after a meal or before bedtime?
– What is the child's schedule?

Para el (la) paciente de pediatría

La criatura, ¿tiene un sarpullido persistente generado por el pañal?
– ¿Cuándo ocurre esto?
– Hay algo que alivie el sarpullido?

¿Cuántos pañales moja la criatura al día?
– ¿Ha cambiado este número recientemente?
    ¿Disminuido?
    ¿Aumentado?

¿Tiene el (la) niño(a) excesiva sed?

¿Cuánto líquido toma por día?

– ¿Qué tipos de líquido?

¿Ha tenido el (la) niño(a) últimamente problemas urinarios?
– ¿Puede Ud. describir el problema?

¿Llora el (la) niño(a) cuando orina?

¿Se ha deteriorado últimamente el control de la vejiga del (de la) niño(a)?

¿Aprendió el (la) niño(a) a sentarse, pararse y hablar a su debido tiempo?

¿Tiene el (la) niño(a) un horario fijo para orinar, por ejemplo, siempre orina después de comer o antes de acostarse?
– ¿Cuál es el horario del (de la) niño(a)?

For the pregnant patient	Para la paciente embarazada

Do you ever have pain when you urinate or pain in the kidney area?
– When did it start?
– How long have you had it?

– What is the pain like?
– What relieves it?

Have you ever been told you had a urinary tract infection?

– When?
– What were your symptoms?
– How was it treated?

How many times do you urinate each day?

How much liquid do you drink each day?

¿Siente Ud. dolor al orinar o en la región del riñón?
– ¿Cuándo comenzó esto?
– ¿Hace cuánto tiempo que lo tiene?
– ¿Cómo es el dolor?
– ¿Qué es lo que lo mitiga?

¿Se le ha diagnosticado alguna vez una infección en el tracto urinario?
– ¿Cuándo?
– ¿Cuáles fueron los síntomas?
– ¿Qué tratamiento se le dió?

¿Cuántas veces orina al día?

¿Cuánto líquido bebe al día?

For the elderly patient	Para el (la) paciente anciano(a)

How much liquid do you drink in the evening?

What types of liquid do you drink in the evening?

Do you ever lose control of your bladder?
– How often does this occur?

– Does this occur suddenly, or do you feel a warning, such as intense pressure?

Do you need help to use the bathroom?

¿Cuánto líquido bebe Ud. en la noche?

¿Qué clase de líquido bebe Ud. en la noche?

¿Ha perdido Ud. control de la vejiga alguna vez?
– ¿Con qué frecuencia ocurre esto?
– ¿Ocurre esto de repente o siente Ud. un aviso, tal como una presión intensa?

¿Necesita ayuda para ir al baño?

Female reproductive system

Current health problems

Bleeding	Sangrado
Have you ever bled between menstrual periods?	**¿Ha tenido alguna vez sangrado entre sus periodos menstruales?**
– When?	– ¿Cuándo?
– How much did you bleed?	– ¿En qué cantidad?
– For how long?	– ¿Por cuánto tiempo?
Have you ever had vaginal bleeding after having sex?	**¿Ha tenido alguna vez sangrado vaginal después de tener relaciones sexuales?**
– When?	– ¿Cuándo?
– How much bleeding did you have?	– ¿Cuánto?
– How long did the bleeding last?	– ¿Por cuánto tiempo?
Have you gone through menopause?	**¿Ya tuvo Ud. la menopausia?**
– How old were you?	– ¿A qué edad?
– When was your last menstrual period?	– ¿Cuándo tuvo Ud. su último periodo menstrual?

Breast changes	Cambios en los senos (las mamas)
Have you noticed any change in your breasts?	**¿Qué cambios ha notado Ud. en los senos?**
How would you describe the change?	**¿Cómo describiría Ud. este cambio?**
– Lump?	– ¿Bultos?
– Thickening?	– ¿Endurecimiento?
– Swelling?	– ¿Hinchazón?
– Skin dimpling?	– ¿Hoyuelos en la piel?
– Pain?	– ¿Dolor?
– Nipple discharge?	– ¿Secreción de los pezones?
When did you first notice the change?	**¿Cuándo notó Ud. el cambio por primera vez?**

155

Female genitalia
Genitales femeninos

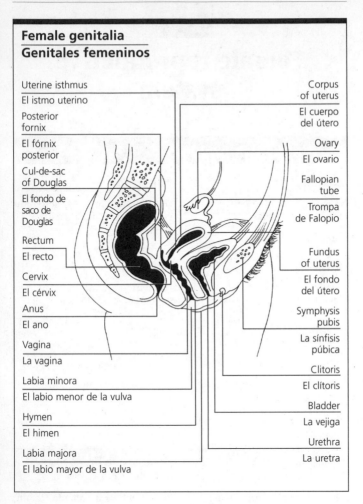

Uterine isthmus
El istmo uterino

Posterior fornix
El fórnix posterior

Cul-de-sac of Douglas
El fondo de saco de Douglas

Rectum
El recto

Cervix
El cérvix

Anus
El ano

Vagina
La vagina

Labia minora
El labio menor de la vulva

Hymen
El himen

Labia majora
El labio mayor de la vulva

Corpus of uterus
El cuerpo del útero

Ovary
El ovario

Fallopian tube
Trompa de Falopio

Fundus of uterus
El fondo del útero

Symphysis pubis
La sínfisis púbica

Clitoris
El clítoris

Bladder
La vejiga

Urethra
La uretra

Has the change improved or worsened?

Have you noticed any change under your arms?
– Describe the change.
– How long ago did you notice it?
– Has it become more obvious lately?

Has any nipple discharge become more noticeable lately?

– Describe the discharge.

¿Se ha mejorado o empeorado?

¿Ha notado Ud. algún cambio en las axilas?
– Descríbalo.
– ¿Hace cuánto tiempo lo notó?
– ¿Se ha vuelto más visible últimamente?

La secreción de los pezones, ¿se ha vuelto más evidente últimamente?
– Describa la secreción.

Female breast
El pecho de la mujer

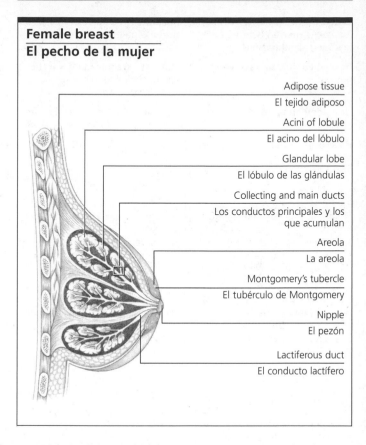

Adipose tissue
El tejido adiposo

Acini of lobule
El acino del lóbulo

Glandular lobe
El lóbulo de las glándulas

Collecting and main ducts
Los conductos principales y los
que acumulan

Areola
La areola

Montgomery's tubercle
El tubérculo de Montgomery

Nipple
El pezón

Lactiferous duct
El conducto lactífero

Does this discharge occur with only one nipple?
– Which nipple?

¿Se produce secreción sólo en un pezón?
– ¿En cuál?

Does the discharge occur spontaneously or when pressure is applied to your nipple?

¿Ocurre la secreción espontáneamente o cuando se aplica presión sobre el pezón?

Do you have any rash or eczema on either nipple?

¿Tiene erupción o eccema en alguno de los pezones?

Menstrual cycle changes

Cambios en el ciclo menstrual

When was the first day of your last menstrual period?

¿Cuándo fue el primer día de su último periodo menstrual?

Was that period similar to your previous periods?

¿Fue ese periodo similar a los periodos anteriores?

When was the first day of the menstrual period before your last menstrual period?

¿Cuándo fue el primer día de su periodo menstrual anterior a ése?

How often do you have your period?
– Are they regular?

¿Con qué frecuencia tiene Ud. sus periodos menstruales?
– ¿Con regularidad?

How long do your periods normally last?

¿Normalmente cuántos días duran sus periodos menstruales?

How would you describe your menstrual flow?
– Heavy?
– Moderate?
– Light?

¿Cómo describiría Ud. su flujo menstrual?
– ¿Fuerte?
– ¿Moderado?
– ¿Ligero?

What color is your menstrual flow?
– Are there any clots?
    Few?
    Moderate number?
    Many?

¿De qué color es su flujo menstrual?
– ¿Contiene coágulos?
    ¿Pocos?
    ¿Un número moderado?
    ¿Muchos?

How many sanitary napkins or tampons do you use each day of your period?
– Has this number changed recently?
    Has it increased?
    Has it decreased?

¿Cuántas toallas higiénicas o tampones usa Ud. cada uno de los días de su periodo?
– ¿Ha cambiado esto últimamente?
    ¿Ha aumentado?
    ¿Ha aminorado?

Pain

Dolor

Do you have pain during your menstual period?
– When does the pain occur?
    Before your periods?
    During your periods?
    After your periods?
    Other?

¿Tiene Ud. dolor?

– ¿Cuándo tiene Ud. el dolor?
    ¿Antes de sus periodos?
    ¿Durante sus periodos?
    ¿Después de sus periodos?
    ¿Otro?

Where do you feel the pain?

¿Dónde siente Ud. el dolor?

Does the pain spread to any other areas of your body?
– Point to where the pain spreads.

¿Se extiende a otra región del cuerpo?
– ¿Me puede Ud. indicar hasta dónde se extiende?

What does the pain feel like?
– Dull and cramping?
– Sharp and stabbing, like a knife?
– Pressure or tightness?
– Burning?

¿Cómo siente Ud. el dolor?
– ¿Sordo y con calambres?
– ¿Agudo y punzante, como un cuchillo?
– ¿Presión o tensión?
– ¿Ardor?

How long does the pain last?
- Is it constant?
- Is it intermittent?

How often does the pain occur?

- Did it start recently?
  When?

What makes the pain better?

What makes the pain worse?

Vaginal discharge

Do you have any vaginal discharge?
- When did it start?
- How long have you had it?

- How much vaginal discharge do you have?
- Describe it.

Does the discharge have an odor?
- Can you describe the odor?

Have you experienced:
- itching?
- burning when you urinate?
- painful intercourse?

- fever?
- chills?
- swelling?

Have you noticed any sores or ulcers?
- Where?

Does your sexual partner have:
- genital sores?
- discharge from his penis?

¿Cuánto tiempo dura el dolor?
- ¿Es constante?
- ¿Es intermitente?

¿Hace cuánto tiempo que Ud. tiene el dolor?
- ¿Comenzó recientemente?
  ¿Cuándo?

¿Qué alivia el dolor?

¿Qué intensifica el dolor?

Secreción vaginal

¿Tiene secreción vaginal?

- ¿Cuándo comenzó?
- ¿Hace cuánto tiempo que Ud. la tiene?
- ¿Cuánta secreción ha notado Ud.?
- Descríbala.

¿La secreción vaginal tiene algún olor?
- ¿Puede Ud. describir el olor?

¿Ha tenido Ud.:
- comezón?
- ardor al orinar?
- dolor cuando tiene relaciones sexuales?
- fiebre?
- escalofríos?
- hinchazón?

¿Ha notado llagas o úlceras?

- ¿Dónde?

¿Su compañero sexual tiene:
- llagas genitales?
- secreción en el pene?

Medical history

How old were you when you had your first menstrual period?

Have you had any discomfort before or during your periods?

¿A qué edad tuvo su primer período menstrual?

¿Ha tenido Ud. malestar antes o durante sus periodos?

Have you gone through menopause?
– How old were you?

¿Ha tenido Ud. la menopausia?

– ¿A qué edad?

During menopause, did you experience:

¿Durante la menopausia tuvo Ud. algunos problemas, tales como:

– hot flashes?
– night sweats?
– excessive weight gain?
– mood swings?
– other signs and symptoms?
    What did you do to relieve them?

– calores?
– sudor nocturno?
– aumento de peso excesivo?
– cambios de humor?
– otro?
    ¿Qué hizo Ud. para aliviarlos?

Has anyone ever told you that something is wrong with your uterus or other reproductive organs?
– Who told you?
– When?
– How was the problem treated?

¿Se le ha dicho que su útero o sus órganos reproductivos tienen un problema?

– ¿Quién se lo dijo?
– ¿Cuándo?
– ¿Cómo se trató el problema?

Have you ever had a sexually transmitted disease or other genital or reproductive system infection?
– What was the problem?
    Chlamydia?
    Gonorrhea?
    Syphilis?
    Other?
– How was it treated?
– Did you develop any complications?
    What were the complications?

¿Ha tenido Ud. alguna vez una enfermedad de transmisión sexual u otra infección genital o del sistema reproductivo?
– ¿Cuál fue el problema?
    ¿Clamidia?
    ¿Gonorrea?
    ¿Sífilis?
    ¿Otra?
– ¿Qué tratamiento se le dió?
– ¿Se presentaron complicaciones?

    ¿Cuáles fueron las complicaciones?

Have you had surgery for a reproductive system problem?

– When?
– What type of surgery?

¿Ha tenido Ud. cirugía a causa de un problema en el sistema reproductivo?
– ¿Cuándo?
– ¿Qué tipo de cirugía?

Have you ever received radiation therapy to your reproductive organs?
– When?
– Why?

¿Se ha aplicado radiación a sus órganos reproductivos?

– ¿Cuándo?
– ¿Por qué?

Have you ever been pregnant?

– How many times?

¿Ha estado Ud. embarazada alguna vez?
– ¿Cuántas veces?

- Have you ever had a miscarriage or an abortion?
   How many times?
- How old were you when you had your children?

Have you ever had any problems during pregnancy?

- What problems did you have?
- When did these problems occur?
   Before the baby was born?

   While you were in labor?
   After the baby was born?
- What treatment did you receive?
- Did any of the problems continue?
   Which ones?
- Were your infants healthy?
   If not, describe the problems they had.
- Did you breast-feed your infants?

Have you ever had problems getting pregnant?
- What treatment did you receive?

Have you ever had breast surgery?
- When?
- Why?

Have you ever had a mammogram?
How old were you when you had your first mammogram?

Do you have regular health checkups, including gynecologic examinations?
- How often?
- When was your last checkup?

When was your last Papanicolaou (PAP) test?
- What was the result?

When was your last mammogram?

- ¿Alguna vez ha tenido Ud. un aborto espontáneo o inducido?
   ¿Cuántas veces?
- ¿A qué edad tuvo Ud. a sus hijos?

¿Ha tenido Ud. alguna vez problemas durante el embarazo?
- ¿Cuáles fueron los problemas?
- ¿Cuándo ocurrió esto?

   ¿Durante el periodo prenatal?
   ¿Durante el parto?
   ¿Después del parto?
- ¿Qué tratamiento se le dió?

- ¿Siguió Ud. teniendo alguno de esos problemas?
   ¿Cuáles?
- ¿Fueron saludables sus hijos?
   ¿Puede Ud. describir los problemas?
- ¿Les dió de mamar a sus hijos?

¿Ha tenido Ud. problemas para concebir?
- ¿Qué tratamiento siguió?

¿Ha tenido Ud. cirugía de los senos?
- ¿Cuándo?
- ¿Por qué razón?

¿Se le ha hecho una mamografía?
- ¿Qué edad tenía Ud. cuando se le hizo la primera?

¿Se realiza habitualmente controles médicos, entre ellos exámenes ginecológicos?
- ¿Con qué frecuencia?
- ¿Cuándo fue su último control?

¿Cuándo se realizó su último análisis de Papanicolau?
- ¿Cómo dieron los resultados?

¿Cuándo se le hizo la última mamografía?

– What was the result?

Do you examine your breasts?
– How often?

– When?

– ¿Cómo dieron los resultados?

¿Examina Ud. sus senos?
– ¿Con qué frecuencia lo hace Ud.?

– ¿Cuándo?

Family history

Has anyone in your family ever had any reproductive problems?
– Difficulty getting pregnant?
– Miscarriage?
– Menstrual difficulties?

– Premature births
– Multiple births?
– Birth defects?
– Difficult pregnancies?

¿Algún miembro de su familia ha tenido alguna vez problemas del sistema reproductivo?
– ¿Dificultad para concebir?
– ¿Aborto espontáneo?
– ¿Dificultades con la menstruación?

– ¿Partos prematuros?
– ¿Nacimiento múltiple?
– ¿Defectos de nacimiento?
– ¿Embarazos difíciles?

Has anyone in your family had:

– high blood pressure?
– diabetes mellitus?
– gestational diabetes?
– obesity?
– heart disease?
– cancer?

¿Algún miembro de su familia ha tenido:
– presión sanguínea alta?
– diabetes mellitus?
– diabetes durante la gestación?
– obesidad?
– enfermedad del corazón?
– cáncer?

Who had this problem?

How was it treated?

Has any member of your immediate family had gynecologic surgery?
– Who?
– What type of surgery?
– Why did she have the surgery?

¿Quién?

¿Qué tratamiento se le dió?

¿Hay algún miembro de su familia cercana que haya tenido cirugía ginecológica?
– ¿Quién?
– ¿Qué tipo de cirugía?
– ¿Cuál fue la razón para la realización la cirugía?

Did your mother or any siblings have breast cancer?

– Who?
– Was the cancer in one or both breasts?
– How was it treated?

¿Su madre o cualquiera de sus hermanas han tenido cáncer de mama?

– ¿Quién?
– ¿Tuvo o tuvieron cáncer en uno o en los dos senos?
– ¿Qué tratamiento se les dió?

Health patterns

Medications	Medicamentos

Do you take any medications?
- Prescription?
- Over-the-counter?
- Home remedies?
- Herbal preparations?
- Other?

¿Toma Ud. medicamentos?
- ¿Con receta?
- ¿De venta libre?
- ¿Remedios caseros?
- ¿Preparados herbales?
- ¿Otro?

Which prescription medications do you take?
- How often do you take them?

¿Qué medicamento de receta toma Ud.?
- ¿Con qué frecuencia los toma?

Which over-the-counter medications do you take?
- How often do you take them?

¿Qué medicamentos de venta libre toma?
- ¿Con qué frecuencia los toma?

Why do you take these medications?

¿Por qué toma Ud. estos medicamentos?

How much of each medication do you take?

¿Cuál es la dosis que Ud. toma de cada uno de estos medicamentos?

How does each medication make you feel?

¿Cómo le hace sentirse cada uno de estos medicamentos?

Are you allergic to any medications?
- Which medications?
- What happens when you have an allergic reaction?

¿Es alérgico(a) a algún medicamento?
- ¿Qué medicamentos?
- ¿Qué le pasa cuando tiene una reacción alérgica?

Are you currently using birth control?
- What kind of birth control do you use?
- How long have you used it?

¿Usa Ud. actualmente algún anticonceptivo?
- ¿De qué tipo?

- ¿Hace cuánto tiempo que lo usa?

Personal habits	Hábitos personales

Do you smoke or chew tobacco?
- What do you smoke?
    Cigarettes?
    Cigars?
    Pipe?
- How long have you smoked or chewed tobacco?

¿Fuma Ud.?

- ¿Qué fuma Ud.?
    ¿Cigarrillos?
    ¿Cigarros (puros)?
    ¿Pipa?
- ¿Hace cuánto tiempo que Ud. fuma o masca tabaco?

– How many cigarettes, cigars, or pipes of tobacco do you smoke each day?
– Did you ever stop?

> For how long?
> What made you decide to stop?
> What method did you use to stop?
> Do you remember why you started again?

– ¿Cuántos cigarrillos, cigarros (puros), o pipas de tabaco fuma Ud. al día?
– ¿Alguna vez dejó Ud. de fumar o mascar tabaco?

> ¿Cuánto tiempo duró?
> ¿Qué lo hizo decidirse a dejar de fumar?
> ¿Qué método usó Ud. para dejar el hábito?
> ¿Recuerda Ud. por qué comenzó a fumar o mascar tabaco otra vez?

If you do not use tobacco now, have you smoked in the past?

Si no consume tabaco actualmente, ¿ha Ud. fumado en el pasado?

Do you drink alcoholic beverages?
– What type?
> Beer?
> Wine?
> Hard liquor?
– How often do you drink alcoholic beverages?
– How many drinks do you have in one day?
> Spread over how much time?

¿Toma Ud. bebidas alcohólicas?
– ¿Qué clase?
> ¿Cerveza?
> ¿Vino?
> ¿Aguardiente?
– ¿Con qué frecuencia toma bebidas alcohólicas?
– ¿Cuántos tragos toma en un día?

> ¿Repartidas en cuánto tiempo?

Sleep patterns

How many hours do you sleep each night?

When you wake up, do you feel rested?

Does your current problem interfere with your sleep pattern?
– How?

Patrones de sueño

¿Cuántas horas duerme por noche?

Cuando se despierta, ¿se siente bien descansado?

Su porblema actual, ¿interfiere con su patrón de sueño?
– ¿Cómo?

Activities

Does your current problem affect your usual activities?
– How?

Actividades

Su problema actual, ¿afecta sus actividades habituales?
– ¿Cómo?

Nutrition

Do you eat a well-balanced diet?

Nutrición

¿Come Ud. una dieta bien equilibrada?

How much fat do you eat?	**¿Qué cantidad de grasa come Ud.?**
Do you follow a special diet?	**¿Sigue Ud. una dieta especial?**
– What type of diet?	– ¿Qué tipo de dieta?
– Who prescribed the diet?	– ¿Quién le recetó la dieta?
What types of fluids do you drink?	**¿Qué tipos de líquidos toma?**
– How much?	– ¿En qué cantidad?

Sexual patterns	**Patrones sexuales**
Are you sexually active?	**¿Tiene Ud. relaciones sexuales actualmente?**
– When was the last time you had sex?	– ¿Cuándo fue la última vez que tuvo relaciones sexuales?
– Do you have sex with more than one partner?	– ¿Tiene Ud. más de un compañero sexual?
Do you do anything to prevent sexually transmitted disease or acquired immunodeficiency syndrome (AIDS)?	**¿Toma Ud. precauciones para no contagiarse de una enfermedad de transmisión sexual o del Síndrome de inmunodeficiencia adquirida (SIDA)?**
– What do you do?	– ¿Qué precauciones toma Ud.?
Do any cultural or religious factors affect what you believe or do about sex and reproduction?	**¿Algunos factores culturales o religiosos afectan sus creencias o hábitos con respecto la sexualidad y la reproducción?**
Do you prefer to have sex with:	**Prefiere tener relaciones sexuales con:**
– men?	– ¿hombres?
– women?	– ¿mujeres?
– both?	– ¿ambos?
Have you noticed any changes in how you feel about sex, how often you have sex, or how your body feels when you have sex?	**¿Ha notado algún cambio en su concepción del sexo, la frecuencia de sus relaciones sexuales o las sensaciones corporales que experimenta al tener relaciones sexuales?**
– What changes?	– ¿Cuáles fueron esos cambios?
– Do these changes affect your emotional and social relationships?	– ¿Estos cambios, sus relaciones emocionales y sociales?

Environment	**Entorno**
Have you ever been exposed to radiation or toxic chemicals?	**¿Ha estado expuesto alguna vez a radiación o a químicos tóxicos?**

– When?	– ¿Cuándo?
– For how long?	– ¿Por cuánto tiempo?
– To what were you exposed?	– ¿A qué estuvo expuesto?

Psychosocial considerations

Coping skills

Habilidad de sobrellevar problemas

Are you under a lot of stress?

¿Diría Ud. que está bajo mucho estrés?

– How long have you been under this much stress?

– ¿Desde hace cuánto tiempo?

What helps you deal with stress?

¿Qué lo ayuda a lidiar con el estrés?

Do you have a close friend or relative who helps you deal with stress?

¿Tiene un amigo íntimo o familiar que lo ayude a lidiar con el estrés?

Roles

Roles

How do your breasts and reproductive organs affect how you feel about yourself?

¿Qué importancia tienen los senos y órganos reproductivos en su manera de verse a usted misma?

Do you have children?

¿Tiene hijos?

How does your problem interfere with your role as a wife and mother?

¿Cómo interfiere su problema con su rol de esposa y madre?

Responsibilities

Responsabilidades

What is your occupation?

¿Cuál es su profesión o trabajo?

What are your typical responsibilities at home?

¿Cuáles son sus responsabilidades típicas en el hogar?

Have your health problems interfered with your responsibilities?

¿Sus problemas de salud han interferido con sus responsabilidades?

– How?

– ¿Cómo?

Developmental considerations

For the pediatric patient

Para la paciente de pediatría

Did the mother use any hormones while she was pregnant?
- What were they?
- When did she take them?
- For how long?

¿Usó la madre hormonas durante el embarazo?

- ¿Cuáles fueron?
- ¿Cuándo tomó las hormonas?
- ¿Por cuánto tiempo?

Did the child have any genitourinary problems at birth?
- How were they treated?

¿Tuvo la criatura problemas genitourinarios?
- ¿Qué tratamiento se les dió?

For the adolescent patient

Para la paciente adolescente

How old were you when you first noticed that you had hair on your pubic area?

¿A qué edad notaste cabello en la región púbica?

How old were you when you first noticed your breasts growing?

¿Cuándo notaste que te crecían los senos?

Have you noticed any moistness on your underpants?

¿Has notado que hay humedad en tu ropa interior?

Have you noticed any blood on your underpants?

¿Has notado alguna mancha de sangre en tu ropa interior?

How old were you when you had your first menstrual period?

¿A qué edad tuviste tu primer período menstrual?

Are you sexually active?

¿Tienes relaciones sexuales actualmente?

- How old were you when you had sex for the first time?

- ¿Qué edad tenías cuando tuviste relaciones sexuales por primera vez?

- Do you ever have pain while having sex?

- ¿Alguna vez sientes dolor durante las relaciones sexuales?

Do you use birth control?
- What do you use?

¿Usa algún anticonceptivo?
- ¿Qué usa?

Do you have any questions or concerns about sexual issues?

¿Tienes alguna pregunta o preocupación sobre temas sexuales?

Is there someone you can talk with about personal issues?

¿Tienes alguien con quien hablar de temas personales?

For the pregnant patient

Have you attented any child-birth classes?

Do you wear a support bra?

Do you plan to breast-feed your baby?

Do you have any concerns about breast-feeding?

Para la paciente embarazada

¿Ha asistido a alguna clase de preparación para el parto?

¿Usa Ud. un sostén de soporte?

¿Piensa Ud. dar de mamar?

¿Se siente Ud. algo ansiosa por dar de mamar?

For the elderly patient

Have you gone through menopause?
– Are you taking hormone thera-py for menopause?
– Have you had any bleeding?

Do you experience hot flushes or hot flashes?
– How often do you have them?

– How do you deal with them?

Have you ever felt vaginal dry-ness, pain, or itching while you were having sex?

Do you have any vaginal bleed-ing?
– How often?
– How much?

Para la paciente anciana

¿Ha tenido Ud. la menopausia?

– ¿Recibe terapia de hormonas para la menopausia?
– ¿Ha tenido Ud. sangrado?

¿Siente Ud. calores?

– ¿Con cuánta frecuencia los tiene?
– ¿Cómo lidia con ellos?

¿Tiene Ud. sequedad, dolor o comezón vaginal durante el coito?

¿Tiene sangrado vaginal?

– ¿Con cuánta frecuencia?
– ¿Cuánta cantidad?

16

Male reproductive system

Current health problems

Changes in appearance

Have you noticed any changes in the color or appearance of the skin on your penis or scrotum?
– What change?
– When did you first notice it?

Are you circumcised?
– Can you easily retract and replace the foreskin?

Cambio de aspecto

¿Ha notado Ud. algún cambio en el color de la piel del pene o del escroto?
– ¿Qué cambio?
– ¿Cuándo lo notó por primera vez?

¿Está usted circuncidado?
– ¿Puede Ud. contraer y reponer el prepucio con facilidad?

Erection difficulties

Do you have any difficulty getting or keeping an erection during sexual activity?

– What type of difficulty?
– How often do you have this problem?
– When did it start?

Do you have erections at other times, such as upon awakening?

Have you ever had pain from an erection?
– Describe the pain.
– How often does it occur?

– What makes it better?

Dificultades en la erección

¿Tiene Ud. alguna dificultad en alcanzar y mantener una erección durante su actividad sexual?
– ¿Qué tipo de dificultad?
– ¿Con qué frecuencia tiene este problema?
– ¿Cuándo comenzó este problema?

¿Tiene Ud. erecciones en otras ocasiones, tal como al despertar?

¿Siente Ud. dolor cuando tiene una erección?
– Describa el dolor.
– ¿Con cuánta frecuencia se produce?
– ¿Qué lo alivia?

Male genitalia
Genitales masculínos

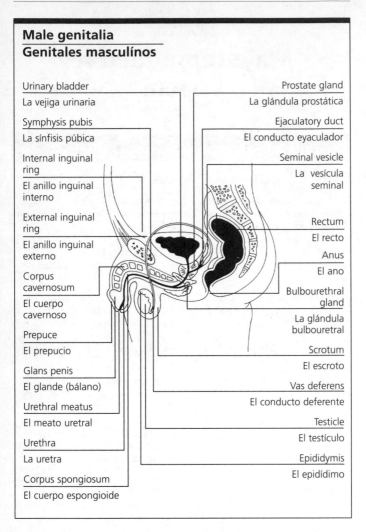

Urinary bladder	Prostate gland
La vejiga urinaria	La glándula prostática
Symphysis pubis	Ejaculatory duct
La sínfisis púbica	El conducto eyaculador
Internal inguinal ring	Seminal vesicle
El anillo inguinal interno	La vesícula seminal
External inguinal ring	Rectum
El anillo inguinal externo	El recto
	Anus
Corpus cavernosum	El ano
El cuerpo cavernoso	Bulbourethral gland
Prepuce	La glándula bulbouretral
El prepucio	Scrotum
Glans penis	El escroto
El glande (bálano)	Vas deferens
Urethral meatus	El conducto deferente
El meato uretral	Testicle
Urethra	El testículo
La uretra	Epididymis
Corpus spongiosum	El epidídimo
El cuerpo espongioide	

Ejaculation difficulties

Do you have any difficulty with ejaculation?
– What type of difficulty?
    Premature ejaculation?
    Delayed ejaculation?

Dificultades en la eyaculación

¿Tiene Ud. alguna dificultad en la eyaculación?
– ¿Qué clase de dificultad?
    ¿Eyaculación precoz?
    ¿Eyaculación retardada?

Retrograde (backward) ejaculation?

¿Eyaculación retrógrada (ingreso de semen en la vejiga al eyacular, en vez de ser expulsado por la uretra)?

Do you ever experience pain during ejaculation?
– How often?

¿Siente Ud. dolor alguna vez durante la eyaculación?
– ¿Con qué frecuencia?

Nocturia

Nocturia

Do you get up during the night to urinate?
– How often?
– When did you start doing this?

¿Se levanta Ud. por la noche para orinar?
– ¿Con qué frecuencia?
– ¿Cuándo comenzó esto?

Do you have:
– urinary frequency?
– hesitancy?
– dribbling?
– pain during urination?
  Describe the problem.
  How often does it occur?

¿Ud.:
– orina con frecuencia?
– tiene vacilación?
– tiene goteo?
– siente dolor al orinar?
  Describa este problema.
  ¿Con qué frecuencia ocurre?

Pain

Dolor

Have you ever had pain in your penis, testes, or scrotum?

– Where?
– When did you have it?

¿Ha tenido alguna vez dolor en el pene, los testículos o el escroto?
– ¿Dónde?
– ¿Cuándo?

How often does the pain occur?

¿Con qué frecuencia siente el dolor?

How long does the pain last?

¿Cuánto dura el dolor?

What does the pain feel like?
– Dull ache?
– Burning?
– Pressure?
– Pulling?
– Sharp and stabbing, like a knife?

¿Cómo siente Ud. el dolor?
– ¿Dolor sordo?
– ¿Ardiente?
– ¿Presión?
– ¿Como si lo estuvieran jalando?
– ¿Agudo y punzante, como un cuchillo?

Does the pain spread?
– Where does it spread?

¿Se extiende el dolor?
– ¿Adónde?

What makes the pain better?

¿Qué es lo que alivia el dolor?

What makes the pain worse?

¿Qué es lo que lo intensifica?

Have you ever felt a lump, painful sore, or tenderness in your groin?

¿Ha notado Ud. un bulto, una llaga dolorosa o sensibilidad excesiva en la ingle?

– When did you feel it?

– ¿Cuándo notó Ud. esto por primera vez?

Penile discharge

Secreción del pene

Have you noticed any discharge from your penis?
– What color is the discharge?
  Yellow?
  Clear?
  Bloody?
  Other?
– What is the consistency of the discharge?
  Thin?
  Thick?

¿Ha notado Ud. alguna secreción del pene?
– ¿De qué color es?
  ¿Amarilla?
  ¿Clara?
  ¿Ensangrentada?
  ¿Otra?
– ¿Cuál es la consistencia de la secreción?
  ¿Fluida?
  ¿Espesa?

Scrotal swelling

Hinchazón del escroto

Have you noticed any swelling in your scrotum?
– When did it start?

¿Ha notado Ud. alguna hinchazón del escroto?
– ¿Cuándo le comenzó?

How would you describe the swelling?
– Constant?
– Intermittent?

¿Cómo describiría Ud. la hinchazón?
– ¿Constante?
– ¿Intermitente?

What makes the swelling better?

¿Qué es lo que hace bajar la hinchazón?

What makes the swelling worse?

¿Qué es lo que agrava la hinchazón?

Is the swelling better or worse than when it started?

¿Ha mejorado o empeorado la hinchazón desde que comenzó?

Medical history

Do you have any children?
– How many?

¿Tiene Ud. hijos?
– ¿Cuántos?

Have you ever had a problem with infertility?
– What was the problem?
– Is it a current concern?

¿Ha tenido Ud. alguna vez algún problema de esterilidad?
– ¿Cuál fue el problema?
– ¿Es esto una preocupación actual?

Have you ever had surgery on the genitourinary tract or for a hernia?

¿Se le practicado alguna vez una cirugía en el tracto genitourinario o a causa de una hernia?

– What kind of surgery did you have?
– When did you have it?
– Why did you have it?

– ¿Qué tipo de cirugía le realizaron?
– ¿Cuándo?
– ¿Por qué?

Did you experience any complications after surgery?
– What were the complications?

– How were they treated?

¿Tuvo Ud. alguna complicación después de la cirugía?
– ¿Cuáles fueron las complicaciones?
– ¿Qué tratamiento se les dió?

Have you ever had an injury to the genitourinary tract?

– What happened?
– When did it happen?
– What symptoms developed as a result?
– How was it treated?

¿Ha tenido Ud. alguna vez una lesión en el tracto genitourinario?
– ¿Qué ocurrió?
– ¿Cuándo ocurrió?
– ¿Qué síntomas se le han desarrollado a causa de esto?
– ¿Cómo fue tratada?

Have you ever been told you had a sexually transmitted disease or other infection in the genitourinary tract?

– What was the problem?
    Chlamydia?
    Gonorrhea?
    Syphilis?
    Other?
– How long did it last?
– How was it treated?
– Did you develop any complications?
– What were the complications?

¿Se le ha diagnosticado alguna vez una enfermedad de transmisión sexual o cualquier otra infección del tracto genitourinario?
– ¿Cuál fue el problema?
    ¿Clamidia?
    ¿Gonorrea?
    ¿Sífilis?
    ¿Otra?
– ¿Cuánto tiempo le duró?
– ¿Qué tratamiento se le dió?
– ¿Surgieron complicaciones?

– ¿Cuáles fueron las complicaciones?

Do you have any other illnesses such as:
– diabetes mellitus?
– heart disease, such as arteriosclerosis?
– neurologic disease, such as multiple sclerosis or amyotrophic lateral sclerosis?
– cancer of the genitourinary tract?
    When?
    How was it treated?

¿Ha tenido Ud. alguno de las siguientes afecciones?
– ¿Diabetes melitus?
– ¿Enfermedad del corazón, tal como arteriosclerosis?
– ¿Enfermedades neurológicas, tal como esclerosis múltiple o esclerosis lateral amiotrófica?
– ¿Cáncer del tracto genitourinario?
    ¿Cuándo?
    ¿Cómo fue tratada?

Do you examine your testes regularly?
– How often?

¿Se examina Ud. los testículos periódicamente?
– ¿Con qué frecuencia?

– Have you been taught how to examine them?

– ¿Se le ha enseñado el procedimiento adecuado?

Do you have a history of undescended testes or an endocrine disorder, such as hypogonadism?

¿Tiene Ud. antecedentes de testículos no descendidos (criptorquidia) o un desorden endocrino, tal como hipogonadismo?

– When was it diagnosed?
– How was it treated?

– ¿Cuándo se le diagnosticó?
– ¿Qué tratamiento se le dió?

Family history

Has anyone in your family had infertility problems?

¿Hay algún miembro de su familia que haya tenido problemas de esterilidad?

– Who?
– How was it treated?

– ¿Quién?
– ¿Qué tratamiento se le dió?

Has anyone in your family had a hernia?

¿Hay algún miembro de su familia que haya tenido una hernia?

– Who?
– How was it treated?

– ¿Quién?
– ¿Qué tratamiento se le dió?

Health patterns

Medications

Medicamentos

Do you take any medications?
– Prescription?
– Over-the-counter?
– Home remedies?
– Herbal preparations?
– Other?

¿Toma Ud. medicamentos?
– ¿Con receta?
– ¿De venta libre?
– ¿Remedios caseros?
– ¿Preparados herbales?
– ¿Otro?

Which prescription drugs do you take?
– How often do you take them?

¿Qué medicamentos de receta toma Ud.?
– ¿Con qué frecuencia los toma Ud.?

Which over-the-counter medications do you take?
– How often do you take them?

¿Qué medicamentos de venta libre toma?
– ¿Con qué frecuencia los toma?

Why do you take these medications?

¿Por qué toma Ud. estos medicamentos?

How much of each medication do you take?

¿Cuál es la dosis para cada uno de los medicamentos?

How does each medication make you feel?

¿Cómo le hace sentirse cada uno de estos medicamentos?

Are you allergic to any medications?
- Which medications?
- What happens when you have an allergic reaction?

¿Es Ud. alérgico a algún medicamento?
- ¿A qué medicamentos?
- ¿Qué le pasa cuando tiene una reacción alérgica?

Personal habits

Do you smoke or chew tobacco?
- What do you smoke?
    Cigarettes?
    Cigars?
    Pipe?
- How long have you smoked or chewed tobacco?
- How many cigarettes, cigars, or pipes of tobacco do you smoke each day?
- How much tobacco do your chew each day?
- Did you ever stop?

    For how long?
    What made you decide to stop?
    What method did you use to stop?
    Do you remember why you started again?

If you do not use tobacco now, have you smoked or chewed tobacco in the past?

Do you drink alcoholic beverages?
- What type?
    Beer?
    Wine?
    Hard liquor?
- How often do you drink alcoholic beverages?
- How many drinks do you have in one day?
    Spread over how much time?

Hábitos personales

¿Fuma Ud. o masca tabaco?
- ¿Qué fuma Ud.?
    ¿Cigarrillos?
    ¿Cigarros (puros)?
    ¿Pipa?
- ¿Hace cuánto tiempo que Ud. fuma o masca tabaco?
- ¿Cuántos cigarrillos, cigarros (puros) o pipas de tabaco fuma Ud. al día?
- ¿Cuánto tabaco masca Ud. al día?
- ¿Alguna vez dejo Ud. de fumar o mascar tabaco?
    ¿Cuánto tiempo duró?
    ¿Qué lo hizo decidirse a dejar de fumar?
    ¿Qué método usó Ud. para dejar el hábito?
    ¿Recuerda Ud. por qué volvió a fumar o mascar tabaco?

Si Ud. no consume tabaco actualmente, ¿ha fumado o mascado tabaco en el pasado?

¿Toma Ud. bebidas alcohólicas?

- ¿Qué clase?
    ¿Cerveza?
    ¿Vino?
    ¿Aguardiente?
- ¿Con qué frecuencia toma bebidas alcohólicas?
- ¿Cuántos tragos toma en un día?
    ¿Repartidas en cuánto tiempo?

Sleep patterns

How many hours do you sleep each night?

When you wake up, do you feel rested?

Does your current problem interfere with your sleep pattern?
– How?

Patrones de sueño

¿Cuántas horas duerme por noche?

Cuando se despierta, ¿se siente bien descansado?

Su problema actual, ¿interfiere con su patrón de sueño?
– Cómo?

Activities

Do you exercise routinely?
– How often?
– What type of exercise do you do?

Do you play sports or engage in any activity that requires heavy lifting or straining?

– How often?

Do you wear any protective or supportive devices, such as a jockstrap, protective cup, or truss?

Actividades

¿Hace Ud. ejercicio habitualmente?
– ¿Con qué frecuencia?
– ¿Qué tipo de ejercicio hace Ud.?

¿Practica deportes o alguna actividad que requiera levantar objetos pesados o hacer esfuerzos intensos?
– ¿Con qué frecuencia?

¿Se pone Ud. un artículo de soporte o de protección, tal como un suspensorio masculino, vaso protector o braguero?

Sexual patterns

Are you sexually active?

– When was the last time you had sex?
– Do you have sex with more than one partner?

Do you do anything to prevent contracting sexually transmitted disease or acquired immunodeficiency syndrome (AIDS)?

– What do you do?

Do you have any difficulties with getting an erection or ejaculating?
– What type of difficulties?

Do any cultural or religious factors affect what you believe

Patrones sexuales

¿Tiene Ud. relaciones sexuales actualmente?
– ¿Cuándo fue la última vez que Ud. tuvo relaciones sexuales?
– ¿Tiene Ud. más de una compañera sexual?

¿Toma Ud. alguna precaución para evitar contagiarse de alguna enfermedad de transmisión sexual o del síndrome de inmunodeficiencia adquirida (SIDA)?
– ¿Cómo se cuida?

¿Tiene Ud. alguna dificultad en la erección o eyaculación?

– ¿Qué clase de dificultad?

¿Hay algunos factores culturales o religiosos que afecten sus

or do about sexuality and reproduction?

Do you prefer to have sex with:

– men?
– women?
– both?

Are you having any sexual problems?
– Describe the problem.
– Is it affecting your emotional and social relationships?

creencias o su práctica con respecto a la sexualidad o procreación?

Prefiere tener relaciones sexuales con:
– ¿hombres?
– ¿mujeres?
– ¿ambos?

¿Tiene Ud. actualmente alguna dificultad sexual?
– Describa el problema.
– ¿Afecta esto sus relaciones emocionales o sociales?

Environment

Have you ever been exposed to radiation or toxic chemicals?
– To what were you exposed?
– When were you exposed?
– How long were your exposed?

Entorno

¿Alguna vez estuvo expuesto a radiación o químicos tóxicos?
– ¿A qué estuvo expuesto?
– ¿Cuándo estuvo Ud. expuesto?
– ¿Por cuánto tiempo estuvo Ud. expuesto?

Psychosocial considerations

Coping skills

Are you under a lot of stress?

– How long have you been under this much stress?

What helps you manage your stress?

Do you have a close friend or relative who helps you deal with stress?

Habilidad de sobrellevar problemas

¿Diría Ud. que está bajo mucho estrés?
– ¿Por cuánto tiempo ha estado muy estresado?

¿Qué lo ayuda a lidiar con el estrés?

¿Tiene un amigo íntimo o familiar que lo ayude a lidiar con el estrés?

Roles

What does it mean to you to be a man?

Do you think you are attractive to others?

Roles

¿Qué significa para usted ser un hombre?

¿Piensa Ud. que otras personas lo consideran atractivo?

Responsibilities

What is your occupation?

Responsabilidades

¿Cuál es su profesión o trabajo?

What are your typical responsibilities at home?
- Have your health problems interfered with your ability to do these things?

    How?

¿Cuáles son sus responsabilidades típicas en el hogar?
- ¿Sus problemas de salud han interferido en su capacidad de cumplir con sus responsabilidades?

    ¿Cómo?

Developmental considerations

For the pediatric patient

Para el paciente de pediatría

Did the mother use any hormones while she was pregnant?
- What hormones did she use?
- When did the mother take them?
- For how long?

¿Usó la madre hormonas durante su embarazo?
- ¿Cuáles fueron?
- ¿Cuándo las tomó la madre?
- ¿Por cuánto tiempo?

Is the child circumcised?

- How do you keep the area clean?

¿Le hicieron la circuncisión al niño?

- ¿Cómo mantiene la higiene en esa zona?

Do you notice any scrotal swelling when the child cries or has a bowel movement?

- How often does this happen?

¿Ha notado Ud. alguna hinchazón escrotal cuando el niño llora o cuando tiene una evacuación intestinal?

- ¿Con qué frecuencia ocurre?

Did the child have genitourinary abnormalities at birth?
- What were they?
- How were they treated?

¿Tuvo el niño anormalidades genitourinarias cuando nació?
- ¿Cuáles?
- ¿Qué tratamiento se les dió?

For the adolescent patient

Para el paciente adolescente

Do you have pubic hair?
- How old were you when you first noticed it?

¿Tienes vello púbico?
- ¿Qué edad tenías cuando lo notaste por primera vez?

Are you sexually active?

- How would you describe your sex life?
- Do you use birth control? What kind?

¿Tienes relaciones sexuales actualmente?
- ¿Cómo describirías tu actividad sexual?
- ¿Usas anticonceptivos? ¿Qué tipo?

Do you have any questions or concerns about sex?

¿Tienes preguntas o inquietudes sobre sexo?

Do you have a support person to talk to about personal issues?

¿Tienes alguien con quien hablar de temas personales?

For the elderly patient

Para el paciente anciano

Have you had any change in how often you have sex or how often you want to have sex?
– What kind of change?

¿Ha tenido Ud. algún cambio en la frecuencia o en el deseo de tener relaciones sexuales?
– ¿Qué clase de cambio?

Have you noticed any changes in your sexual performance?
– What kind of changes?

¿Ha notado Ud. algún cambio en su desempeño sexual?
– ¿Qué clase de cambio?

17

Neurologic system

Current health problems

Auditory changes

How well do you hear?

Have you noticed any change in your hearing?
- What kind of change?
- Does it affect one ear? Which one?
- When did it start?

Do you wear a hearing aid?
- In which ear?
- Does it help?
- Do you wear it all the time?

Difficulty speaking

Have you ever had trouble speaking?
- What happened when you tried to speak?
- When did this happen?
- How long did it last?

Do you have difficulty expressing the words you are thinking?
- What happens?
- When did you first notice this?

Difficulty swallowing

Do you have any trouble swallowing?
- How would you describe the problem?
- When did it start?

Cambios en la audición

¿Cómo está su audición?

¿Ha notado Ud. algún cambio en su audición?
- ¿Qué tipo de cambio?
- ¿Le afecta un oído? ¿Cuál?
- ¿Cuándo empezó?

¿Usa Ud. un audífono?
- ¿En qué oído?
- ¿Le ayuda?
- ¿Lo usa Ud. todo el tiempo?

Dificultades en el habla

¿Tiene Ud. dificultad para hablar?
- ¿Qué ocurría cuando trataba de hablar?
- ¿Cuándo notó Ud. esto por primera vez?
- ¿Cuánto duró?

¿Tiene dificultad en expresar las palabras que Ud. piensa?

- ¿Qué ocurre?
- ¿Cuándo notó Ud. esto por primera vez?

Dificultad para tragar

¿Tiene Ud. dificultad para tragar?
- ¿Cómo la describiría Ud.?
- ¿Cuándo comenzó?

Brain
El cerebro

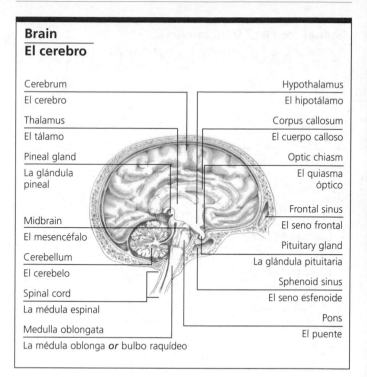

Cerebrum	Hypothalamus
El cerebro	El hipotálamo
Thalamus	Corpus callosum
El tálamo	El cuerpo calloso
Pineal gland	Optic chiasm
La glándula pineal	El quiasma óptico
Midbrain	Frontal sinus
El mesencéfalo	El seno frontal
Cerebellum	Pituitary gland
El cerebelo	La glándula pituitaria
Spinal cord	Sphenoid sinus
La médula espinal	El seno esfenoide
Medulla oblongata	Pons
La médula oblonga *or* bulbo raquídeo	El puente

Do you have problems swallowing everything you eat and drink?
– What foods or drinks give you trouble?

¿Tiene Ud. problemas para tragar toda clase de alimentos y bebidas?
¿Qué alimentos o bebidas le causan dificultad?

Dizziness

Do you have problems with your balance?

Do you have dizzy spells?
– How often do they occur?
– Are they associated with any activity?
– How long do they last?

When did you first start having dizzy spells?

What makes them better?

What makes them worse?

Mareos

¿Tiene Ud. problemas de equilibrio?

¿Tiene Ud. accesos de mareo?
– ¿Con qué frecuencia ocurren?
– ¿Están relacionados con alguna actividad?
– ¿Cuánto tiempo duran?

¿Cuándo notó Ud. estos mareos por primera vez?

¿Qué es lo que los mitiga?

¿Qué es lo que los intensifica?

Spinal cord and spinal nerves
La columna vertebral y los nervios espinales

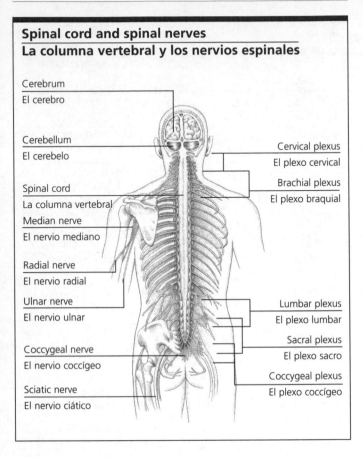

Cerebrum
El cerebro

Cerebellum
El cerebelo

Spinal cord
La columna vertebral

Median nerve
El nervio mediano

Radial nerve
El nervio radial

Ulnar nerve
El nervio ulnar

Coccygeal nerve
El nervio coccígeo

Sciatic nerve
El nervio ciático

Cervical plexus
El plexo cervical

Brachial plexus
El plexo braquial

Lumbar plexus
El plexo lumbar

Sacral plexus
El plexo sacro

Coccygeal plexus
El plexo coccígeo

Have they gotten worse since they first started?

¿Han empeorado desde la primera vez que se presentaron?

Fainting

Have you ever fainted or blacked out, even if only for a few moments?
– When did this happen?
– How long did the episode last?

– Has it happened more than once?

Did anything happen before you fainted?
– What happened?

Desmayos

¿Alguna vez se ha desmayado o perdido la conciencia momentáneamente?
– ¿Cuándo ocurrió esto?
– ¿Cuánto tiempo duró el incidente?
– ¿Le ha ocurrido más de una vez?

¿Le ocurrió algo antes que se desmayara?
– ¿Qué pasó?

Do you have difficulty recalling blocks of time?	**¿Tiene Ud. dificultad para recordar periodos de tiempo?**

Headaches / Dolores de cabeza

Do you have headaches?
- How often do they occur?
- How long do they last?

¿Tiene Ud. dolores de cabeza?
- ¿Con qué frecuencia?
- ¿Cuánto tiempo duran?

Do the headaches seem to follow a pattern?
- What kind of pattern?

¿Siguen los dolores de cabeza un patrón?
- ¿Qué clase de patrón?

When do you usually get a headache?
- Early morning?
- During the day?
- At night?
- At certain times of the month?
- In certain types of weather?

¿Por lo general, a qué hora le dan los dolores de cabeza?
- ¿Temprano por la mañana?
- ¿Durante el día?
- ¿Por la noche?
- ¿En cierta parte del mes?
- ¿Con ciertos cambios del tiempo?

What kind of pain do you feel when you have a headache?
- Sharp, stabbing?
- Dull ache?
- Throbbing?
- Pressure?
- Other?

¿Qué tipo de dolor de cabeza tiene Ud.?
- ¿Agudo o punzante?
- ¿Sordo?
- ¿Palpitante?
- ¿De presión?
- ¿Otro?

Where do you feel the pain?
- Across your forehead?
- Behind your eyes?
- Along your temples?

- In the back of your head?

¿Dónde siente Ud. el dolor?
- ¿A lo largo de la frente?
- ¿Detrás de los ojos?
- ¿En la región lateral de la cabeza?
- ¿En la parte de atrás de la cabeza?

Do you have any other signs or symptoms when you have a headache?
- What are they?
  Nausea?
  Vomiting?
  Stiff neck?
  Blurred vision?
  Sensitivity to light?
  Other?

¿Tiene Ud. otros síntomas junto con los dolores de cabeza?

- ¿Cuáles son?
  ¿Náuseas?
  ¿Vómito?
  ¿Tortícolis?
  ¿Visión borrosa?
  ¿Sensibilidad a la luz?
  ¿Otro?

What makes your headache better?

¿Qué hace Ud. para mitigar el dolor de cabeza?

What makes your headache worse?

¿Qué intensifica su dolor de cabeza?

Memory changes

Have you noticed a change in your ability to remember things?
– How would you describe this change?
    Problems remembering things that happened recently?
    Problems remembering things that happened a long time ago?

Have you noticed any change in your mental alertness or ability to concentrate?
– What kind of change?
– When did it begin?

Do you have trouble following conversations or television programs?

– When did this problem start?

Do you have difficulty concentrating on activities that you once enjoyed, such as reading or watching movies?
– When did this problem start?

Muscle coordination

How would you rate your muscle strength?

Have you recently noticed any change in your strength?
– What kind of change?
– When did it start?

How would you rate your muscle coordination?

Do you often drop things?

– How often?
– When did you begin dropping things?

Cambios en la memoria

¿Ha notado Ud. algún cambio en su habilidad de recordar cosas?
– ¿Cómo describiría Ud. este cambio?
    ¿Problemas para recordar hechos recientes?

    ¿Problemas para recordar hechos lejanos?

¿Ha notado Ud. algún cambio en su agudeza mental o en su habilidad de concentrarse?
– ¿Qué tipo de cambio?
– ¿Cuándo comenzó el cambio?

¿Tiene Ud. dificultad para seguir el hilo de una conversación o un programa de televisión?
– ¿Cuándo comenzó este problema?

¿Tiene Ud. dificultad para concentrarse en actividades que anteriormente gozaba, tal como leer o mirar películas?
– ¿Cuándo comenzó este problema?

Coordinación muscular

¿Cómo clasificaría Ud. su fuerza muscular?

¿Ha notado Ud. últimamente algún cambio en su fuerza?
– ¿Qué tipo de cambio?
– ¿Cuándo comenzó?

¿Cómo clasificaría Ud. su coordinación muscular?

¿Se le caen con frecuencia objetos de la mano?
– ¿Con qué frecuencia?
– ¿Cuándo comenzaron a caérsele las cosas?

Do you have difficulty walking?

– What kind of difficulty?
  Loss of balance?
  Staggering gait?
  Shuffling gait?
  Weakness?
  Loss of sensation?
– Do you use anything to help you walk?
  What do you use?

¿Tiene Ud. dificultad para caminar?

– ¿Qué tipo de dificultad?
  ¿Pérdida de equilibrio?
  ¿Camina tambaleándose?
  ¿Arrastra los pies al caminar?
  ¿Debilidad?
  ¿Pérdida de sensación?
– ¿Usa Ud. algún aparato de apoyo?
  ¿Qué usa Ud.?

Muscle spasms

Do your hands, arms, or legs shake or tremble?

– When did you first notice this?

– Has it gotten worse or improved?
– How often does it occur?

– How long does it last?

When you shake or tremble do you notice:
– numbness?
– tingling?
– feeling of cold?

What makes it better?

What makes it worse?

Espasmos musculares

¿Tiene Ud. temblores o espasmos musculares en las manos, los brazos o las piernas?

– ¿Cuándo los notó Ud. por primera vez?
– ¿Han empeorado o mejorado?

– ¿Con qué frecuencia se producen?
– ¿Cuánto duran?

¿Tiene Ud. _____ junto con los temblores o espasmos?
– ¿Adormecimiento?
– ¿Hormigueo?
– ¿Sensación de frío?

¿Qué los alivia?

¿Qué los intensifica?

Numbness

Have you noticed any change in your ability to feel textures?

– What type of change?

Do you have any numbness, tingling, or other unusual sensations?
– When did you first notice this?

– Where is it?

What makes it better?

What makes it worse?

Adormecimiento

¿Ha notado Ud. algún cambio en su habilidad de percibir texturas?

– ¿Qué tipo de cambio?

¿Siente Ud. adormecimiento, hormigueo u otras sensaciones raras?
– ¿Cuándo notó Ud. esto por primera vez?
– ¿Dónde las localiza Ud.?

¿Qué las alivia?

¿Qué las intensifica?

Visual changes

How well do you see?

Do you wear eyeglasses or contact lenses?
– Why do you need them?
  Near-sightedness?
  Far-sightedness?
  Reading?
  Other problem?

Do you have:

– blurred vision?
– double vision?
– visual disturbances, such as blind spots?

Cambios en la vista

¿Cómo calificaría su visión?

¿Usa anteojos o lentes de contacto?
– ¿Por qué los necesita Ud.?
  ¿Miopía?
  ¿Hipermetropía?
  ¿Para leer?
  ¿Otro problema?

¿Tiene Ud. alguno de los siguientes problemas?
– ¿Visión borrosa?
– ¿Visión doble?
– ¿Otros trastornos visuales, tal como ver puntos negros?

Medical history

Have you ever had a head injury?
– When?
– Describe what happened.
– How was it treated?
– Do you have current problems as a result of the injury?

Have you ever been treated by a neurologist or neurosurgeon?

– When?
– Why?

Have you ever had a seizure?

– When?
– Was this the first time you had a seizure?
– What happened before the seizure?
– What happened during the seizure?
– How long did the seizure last?

– Can you remember anything about the seizure?

How often do you have seizures?

¿Ha tenido Ud. alguna vez una lesión en la cabeza?
– ¿Cuándo?
– ¿Describa lo que sucedió?
– ¿Cómo fue tratada?
– ¿Le quedan efectos perdurables de la lesión?

¿Ha estado Ud. alguna vez bajo el cuidado de un neurólogo o de un neurocirujano?
– ¿Cuándo?
– ¿Por qué?

¿Alguna vez ha tenido convulsiones?
– ¿Cuándo?
– ¿Fue ésa la primera vez que Ud. tuvo convulsiones?
– ¿Qué pasó antes de las convulsiones?
– ¿Qué le pasó durante las convulsiones?
– ¿Cuánto tiempo duraron las convulsiones?
– ¿Tiene algún recuerdo de las convulsiones?

¿Con cuánta frecuencia sufre convulsiones?

Have you ever had a stroke?

– When did it happen?
– What happened to you when you had the stroke?
– Was this the first time that you had a stroke?
– What treatment did you receive for the stroke?
– Do you you still experience problems as a result of the stroke?

Do you have any other illnesses, such as:
– diabetes mellitus?
– heart disease?
– high blood pressure?

¿Ha tenido Ud. alguna vez un derrame cerebral?

– ¿Cuándo lo tuvo?
– ¿Qué le pasó cuando tuvo el derrame cerebral?
– ¿Fue ésta la primera vez que Ud. tuvo un derrame cerebral?
– ¿Qué tratamiento recibió Ud. para el derrame cerebral?
– ¿Aún tiene problemas a raíz del derrame cerebral?

¿Tiene alguna otra enfermedad, como:
– diabetes mellitus?
– enfermedad cardiaca?
– hipertensión?

Family history

Have any family members had a neurologic disease, such as a brain tumor, degenerative disease, or senility?

– Which relative?
– What was the problem?
– How was it treated?

Have any of your immediate family members (mother, father, or siblings) had:

– high blood pressure?
– stroke?
– diabetes mellitus?
– heart disease?
– seizure disorder?
– migraine headaches?

¿Hay algún miembro de su familia que haya tenido una enfermedad neurológica, tal como tumor cerebral, enfermedad degenerativa o senilidad?

– ¿Qué pariente?
– ¿Cuál fue el problema?
– ¿Qué tratamiento se le dió?

¿Hay algún miembro de su familia cercana (madre, padre o hermano[a]) que haya tenido alguno de los siguientes problemas?

– ¿Alta presión sanguínea?
– ¿Derrame cerebral?
– ¿Diabetes melitus?
– ¿Enfermedad del corazón?
– ¿Problemas de convulsiones?
– ¿Migrañas?

Health patterns

Medications

Do you take any medications?
– Prescription?
– Over-the-counter?
– Home remedies?

Medicamentos

¿Toma Ud. medicamentos?
– ¿Con receta?
– ¿De venta libre?
– ¿Remedios caseros?

– Herbal preparations?
– Other?

Which prescription drugs do you take?
– How often do you take them?

Which over-the-counter medications do you take?
– How often do you take them?

Why do you take these medications?

How much of each medication do you take?

How does each medication make you feel?

Are you allergic to any medications?
– Which medications?
– What happens when you have an allergic reaction?

Personal habits

Do you smoke or chew tobacco?
– What do you smoke?
    Cigarettes?
    Cigars?
    Pipe?
– How long have you smoked or chewed tobacco?
– How many cigarettes, cigars, or pipes of tobacco do you smoke each day?
– How much tobacco do you chew each day?
– Did you ever stop?

    For how long?
    What made you decide to stop?
    What method did you use to stop?
    Do you remember why you started again?

– ¿Preparados herbales?
– ¿Otro?

¿Qué medicamentos de receta toma Ud.?
– ¿Con qué frecuencia los toma?

¿Qué medicamentos de venta libre toma Ud.?
– ¿Con qué frecuencia los toma Ud.?

¿Por qué toma estos medicamentos?

¿Cuál es la dosis para cada uno de estos medicamentos?

¿Cómo le hace sentirse a Ud. cada uno de estos medicamentos?

¿Es Ud. alérgico(a) a algún medicamento?
– ¿A qué medicamentos?
– ¿Qué le pasa cuando tiene una reacción alérgica?

Hábitos personales

¿Fuma Ud. o masca tabaco?

– ¿Qué fuma Ud.?
    ¿Cigarrillos?
    ¿Cigarros (puros)?
    ¿Pipa?
– ¿Hace cuánto tiempo que Ud. fuma o masca tabaco?
– ¿Cuántos cigarrillos, cigarros (puros) o pipas de tabaco fuma Ud. al día?
– ¿Cuánto tabaco masca Ud. al día?
– ¿Alguna vez dejó Ud. de fumar o mascar tabaco?
    ¿Por cuánto tiempo?
    ¿Qué lo hizo decidirse a dejar de fumar o mascar tabaco?
    ¿Qué método usó Ud. para dejar el hábito?
    ¿Recuerda Ud. por qué comenzó a fumar o mascar tabaco otra vez?

If you do not use tobacco now, have you smoked or chewed tobacco in the past?

Si Ud. no consume tabaco actualmente, ¿ha fumado o mascado tabaco en el pasado?

Do you drink alcoholic beverages?
– What type?
  Beer?
  Wine?
  Hard liquor?
– How often do you drink alcoholic beverages?
– How many drinks do you have in one day?
  Spread over how much time?

¿Toma Ud. bebidas alcohólicas?

– ¿Qué clase de bebidas?
  ¿Cerveza?
  ¿Vino?
  ¿Aguardiente?
– ¿Con qué frecuencia toma bebidas alcohólicas?
– ¿Cuántos tragos toma en un día?
  ¿Repartidas en cuánto tiempo?

Sleep patterns

How many hours do you sleep each night?

When you wake up, do you feel rested?

Does your current problem interfere with your sleep pattern?
– How?

Patrones de sueño

¿Cuántas horas duerme Ud. cada noche?

¿Se siente Ud. descansado a la mañana siguiente?

Su problema actual, ¿interfiere con su patrón de sueño?
– ¿Cómo?

Activities

What do you do with your spare time?

How much energy do you usually have?

Do you enjoy reading or listening to music?

Do you need to rest during the day?

Do you have more strength at certain times of the day?
– At what times?

Actividades

¿Qué hace Ud. en su tiempo libre?

¿Cuánta energia tiene habitualmente?

¿Le gusta leer o escuchar música?

¿Necesita Ud. descansar durante el día?

¿Tiene mayor fuerza en determinados momentos del día?
– ¿En qué momentos ?

Nutrition

Are you on a special kind of diet?
– What kind of diet?

How much water do you drink each day?

Nutrición

¿Sigue alguna dieta especial?

– ¿Qué tipo de dieta?

¿Cuánta agua bebe por día?

Sexual patterns

Have you noticed any change in your sex life?
– What type of change?

Have you noticed a change in your sex drive?
– Has it increased or decreased?

Environment

Are you exposed to any poisons or chemicals at home or at work?
– To what poisons or chemicals are you exposed?
– How long have you been exposed to them?

At work, do you perform any strenuous or repetitive activities?
– What type of activities?

Do you sit, stand, or walk at your job?

Patrones sexuales

¿Ha notado Ud. algún cambio en su vida sexua?
– ¿Qué tipo de cambio?

¿Ha notado Ud. algún cambio en su libido?
– ¿Ha aumentado o disminuido?

Entorno

¿Está Ud. expuesto a tóxicos o productos químicos en su casa o en su trabajo?
– ¿A qué tóxicos o químicos está expuesto?
– ¿Hace cuánto que está expuesto?

¿En su trabajo, realiza Ud. actividades que son arduas o reiterativas?
– ¿Qué tipo de actividades?

¿Se sienta, se para o camina Ud. mientras desempeña su trabajo?

Psychosocial considerations

Coping skills

What would you consider to be a stressful situation?

How would you handle a stressful situation?

Roles

Has your condition made you feel different about yourself?

– How?

Can you do the things for yourself that you want to do?

How has your illness or disability affected the way members of your family feel?

Habilidad de sobrellevar problemas

¿Qué situación le parecería estresante?

¿Cómo manejaría tal situación?

Roles

Su problema, ¿ha cambiado la manera en la que se siente respecto de usted mismo(a)?
– ¿Cómo?

¿Puede hacer usted mismo(a) las cosas que desea?

¿Cómo ha afectado emocionalmente a los miembros de su familia su enfermedad o discapacidad?

Responsibilities

Can you fulfill your usual responsibilities at home?

– If not, who does them?

What financial impact has your illness or disability had on your family?

Responsabilidades

¿Puede cumplir sus responsabilidades habituales en su hogar?

– De no ser así ¿quién ha asumido esas responsabilidades?

¿Económicamente, cómo ha afectado su enfermedad o discapacidad a los miembros de su familia?

Developmental considerations

For the pediatric patient

Does your family have a history of genetic or familial disorders, such as epilepsy, cerebral palsy, or Down syndrome?

Was the infant full-term or premature?
– How premature was the infant?

Was the infant's birth difficult?

Were medications used during the infant's birth?

How did the infant look right after the birth?

During the first month after birth, did the infant have any problems with sucking or swallowing?

Did the infant have any medical problems, such as high bilirubin levels or a positive test for phenylketonuria?

Has the child received all recommended immunizations?

Para el (la) paciente de pediatría

¿Tiene Ud. antecedentes familiares médicos de trastornos genéticos o familiares, tal como epilepsia, parálisis cerebral o síndrome de Down?

¿Nació el (la) infante(a) a término o fue prematuro?
– ¿Cuán prematuro fue el nacimiento del (de la) infante(a)?

¿Fue difícil el parto?

¿Se le dieron medicamentos durante el parto?

¿Qué semblante tenía el (la) infante(a) inmediatamente después del parto?

¿Al mes de haber nacido, tuvo el (la) infante(a) problemas de amamantamiento o deglución?

¿Tuvo problemas médicos, tal como alto nivel de bilirrubina o un análisis positivo de fenilcetonuria?

¿Ha tenido la criatura todas las vacunas que se le han recomendado?

Has the child recently been exposed to measles, chickenpox, or mumps?

¿Ha estado la criatura expuesta recientemente al sarampión, la varicela o las paperas?

Has the child had any illnesses or injuries?
– What type of injury or illness?
– Did the child receive any medications to treat the illness or injury?

¿Ha tenido la criatura alguna enfermedad o lesión?
– ¿De qué tipo?
– ¿Se dió a la criatura algún medicamento para tratar la enfermedad o la lesión?

Has the child reached developmental milestones, such as sitting up or walking, at the expected age?

¿Ha alcanzado la criatura hitos en el desarrollo, tal como sentarse o andar a la edad esperada?

Has the child lost the ability to do things he used to be able to do?

¿Ha perdido la criatura algunas funciones que había dominado previamente?

Does the child go to school?

¿El (la) niño(a) asiste al colegio?

– How is the child's progress in school?

– ¿Cómo va el progreso del (de la) niño(a) en el colegio?

Does the child have any favorite activities, such as roller skating, bicycling, or jumping rope?

¿Tiene actividades favoritas el (la) niño(a), tal como patinar, andar en bicicleta o saltar la soga?

Has the child had any broken bones or head injuries?

¿El (la) niño(a) se ha quebrado algún hueso o ha tenido lesiones en la cabeza?

– How would you describe these injuries?

– ¿Cómo las describiría Ud.?

For the pregnant patient

Para la paciente embatazada

During pregnancy, have you been exposed to:
– X-rays?
– viruses, such as toxoplasmosis, rubella, cytomegalovirus, or herpes simplex?

Durante su embarazo, ¿ha estado expuesta a:
– rayos X?
– virus, como toxoplasmosis, rubeola, citomegalovirus o herpes simple?

Have you been sick or injured?

¿Ha estado enferma o lesionada?

– In what way?

– ¿Cómo?

Have you had surgery?
– What for?

¿Ha sido operada?
– ¿Por qué razón?

Do you drink or smoke?

¿Bebe o fuma?

For the elderly patient	Para el (la) paciente anciano(a)

Is it harder to get around than it used to be?

¿Le resulta más dificil mobilizarse que antes?

Do you trip or fall more frequently than you used to?
– How often?

¿Se tropieza o se cae Ud. con más frecuencia?
– ¿Con qué frecuencia?

How would you describe the way you walk?
– Has it changed?
– When did it change?
– Have you developed tremors?

¿Cómo describiría Ud. su forma de andar?
– ¿Ha cambiado?
– ¿Cuándo cambió?
– ¿Tiene usted temblores?

Have you noticed any change in your memory or thinking abilities, vision, hearing, or sense of smell or taste?
– What is the change?
– When did it start?

¿Ha notado Ud. algún cambio en la memoria o habilidad de pensar, visión, oído o sentido del olfato o del gusto?
– ¿En qué consiste el cambio?
– ¿Cuándo comenzó?

18

Musculoskeletal system

Current health problems

Impaired movement

When did you first notice your movement was impaired?

Do you have a problem with:
– raising your arm?
– turning your head?
– kneeling?
– bending over?
– other movements?

Do you think your ability to move is limited by pain or something else?
– What do you think might be causing this problem?

Does anything make it easier for you to move?
– What?

Have you noticed any other signs or symptoms, such as fever, rash, numbness, tingling, or swelling?

Pain

Are you having any pain?
– Point to the area where you feel pain.

How long have you had the pain?

Do you know what causes the pain?

Trastorno del movimiento

¿Cuándo notó Ud. por primera vez un trastorno del movimiento?

¿Tiene problemas al:
– levantar el brazo?
– voltear la cabeza?
– arrodillarse?
– agacharse?
– otros movimientos?

¿Piensa Ud. que su movimiento es limitado por el dolor o por otro motivo?
– ¿Qué otro motivo piensa Ud. que podría ser la causa de este problema?

¿Hay algo que le facilite el movimiento?
– ¿Qué?

¿Ha notado Ud. algún otro síntoma, tal como fiebre, erupción, adormecimiento, hormigueo o hinchazón?

Dolor

¿Tiene Ud. dolor actualmente?
– ¿Me puede indicar dónde siente Ud. el dolor?

¿Hace cuánto tiempo que Ud. tiene este dolor?

¿Conoce la causa del dolor?

Does the pain occur at any specific time?
- When?
    In the early morning?
    During the day?
    After you do certain things?

    At night?
    While you are sleeping?

How would you describe the pain?
- Dull ache?
- Burning?
- Sharp and stabbing, like a knife?
- Throbbing?
- Pressure?
- Constant?
- Intermittent?

When you have this pain, do you have pain anywhere else?

- Where?
- Does this pain feel like the other pain?

What makes the pain better?

What makes the pain worse?

When you have the pain, do you have any:
- tingling?
- burning?
- prickling?
- numbness?

¿Le viene el dolor a una hora específica?
- ¿Cuándo?
    ¿Temprano por la mañana?
    ¿Durante el curso del día?
    ¿Después de hacer determinadas actividades?
    ¿Por la noche?
    ¿Mientras Ud. duerme?

¿Cómo describiría Ud. el dolor?

- ¿Dolor sordo?
- ¿Ardor?
- ¿Agudo y punzante, como un cuchillo?
- ¿Pulsante?
- ¿Presión?
- ¿Constante?
- ¿Intermitente?

Cuando Ud. tiene este dolor, ¿siente al mismo tiempo dolor en otro lugar?
- ¿Dónde?
- ¿Es el dolor de esta región del mismo tipo que el otro?

¿Qué alivia el dolor?

¿Qué intensifica el dolor?

Cuando siente dolor, ¿tiene:

- hormigueo?
- ardor?
- picazón?
- adormecimiento?

Stiffness	Rigidez

When did your first feel the stiffness?

How would you describe the stiffness?
- Constant?
- Intermittent?

Does the stiffness occur at any specific time?
- When?
    Early morning?
    During the day?

¿Cuándo empezó a sentir rigidez?

¿Cómo describiría Ud. la rigidez?
- ¿Constante?
- ¿Intermitente?

¿Siente Ud. la rigidez a una hora en particular?
- ¿Cuándo?
    ¿Por la mañana temprano?
    ¿Durante el curso del día?

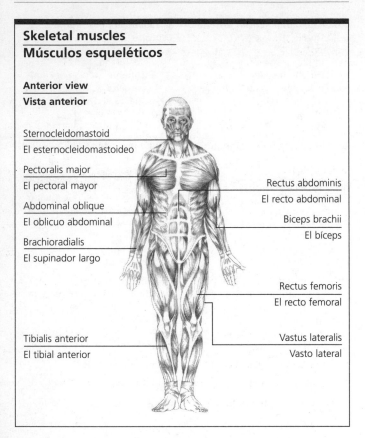

Skeletal muscles
Músculos esqueléticos

Anterior view
Vista anterior

Sternocleidomastoid
El esternocleidomastoideo

Pectoralis major
El pectoral mayor

Abdominal oblique
El oblicuo abdominal

Brachioradialis
El supinador largo

Tibialis anterior
El tibial anterior

Rectus abdominis
El recto abdominal

Biceps brachii
El bíceps

Rectus femoris
El recto femoral

Vastus lateralis
Vasto lateral

After you do certain things?	¿Después de hacer determinadas actividades?
At night?	¿Por la noche?
While you are sleeping?	¿Mientras Ud. duerme?

Do you feel more stiffness than you used to?

¿Ha aumentado la rigidez desde que empezó?

Do you have pain with the stiffness?

¿Tiene Ud. dolor junto con la rigidez?

– What is the pain like?
    Dull ache?
    Burning?
    Sharp and stabbing, like a knife?
    Throbbing?
    Pressure?

– ¿Cómo es el dolor?
    ¿Dolor sordo?
    ¿Ardor?
    ¿Agudo y punzante, como un cuchillo?
    ¿Pulsante?
    ¿Presión?

Do you sometimes hear a grating sound or feel a grating sen-

¿Hay veces que Ud. oye o siente un chirrido como si los huesos

Skeletal muscles
Músculos esqueléticos

Posterior view
Vista posterior

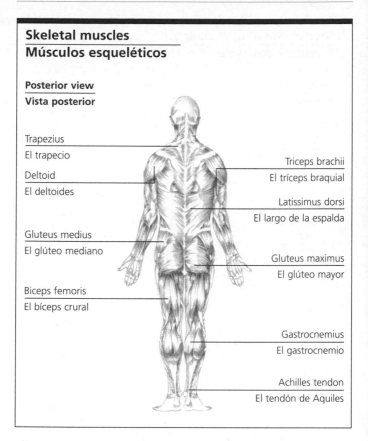

Trapezius
El trapecio

Deltoid
El deltoides

Gluteus medius
El glúteo mediano

Biceps femoris
El bíceps crural

Triceps brachii
El tríceps braquial

Latissimus dorsi
El largo de la espalda

Gluteus maximus
El glúteo mayor

Gastrocnemius
El gastrocnemio

Achilles tendon
El tendón de Aquiles

sation as if your bones are scraping together?

What have you done to try to reduce the stiffness?

Swelling

When did you first notice the swelling?

Did you hurt this part of your body?

Is the area tender?

Does the skin in this area ever look red or feel hot?

What have you done to try to reduce the swelling?

se estuvieran raspando los unos contra los otros?

¿Qué métodos ha probado Ud. para disminuir la rigidez?

Hinchazón

¿Cuándo notó Ud. la hinchazón por primera vez?

¿Se lastimó esa parte del cuerpo?

¿Está adolorida esta región?

¿Parece a veces que la epidermis está enrojecida y caliente?

¿Qué método ha probado Ud. para reducir la hinchazón?

Bones of the human skeleton
Los huesos del esqueleto humano

Anterior view
Vista anterior

Skull
El cráneo

Frontal
El hueso frontal
Temporal
El hueso temporal

Mandible
La mandíbula

Clavicle
La clavícula

Humerus
El húmero

Sternum
El esternón

Ribs
Las costillas

Ulna
La ulna

Radius
El radio

Pubis
El pubis

Carpals
Los huesos del carpo

Femur
El fémur

Phalanges
Las falanges
del dedo

Patella
La rótula

Metacarpals
Los huesos del
metacarpo

Tibia
La tibia

Fibula
El peroné

Metatarsals
El metatarso

Tarsals
El tarso

Phalanges
Las falanges

– Have you used heat?   – ¿Le ha aplicado calor?
– Have you used ice?   – ¿Le ha aplicado hielo?

Posterior view
Vista posterior

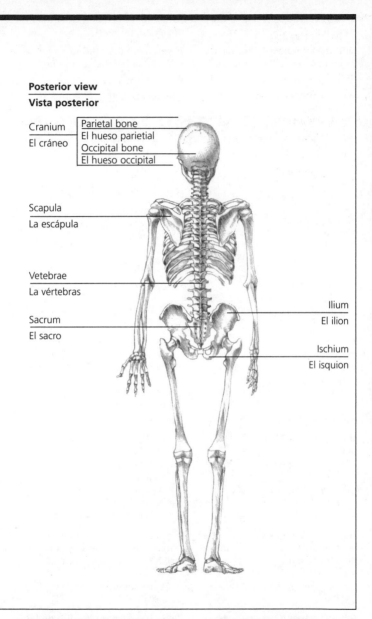

Cranium
El cráneo

Parietal bone
El hueso parietial
Occipital bone
El hueso occipital

Scapula
La escápula

Vetebrae
La vértebras

Sacrum
El sacro

Ilium
El ilion

Ischium
El isquion

Weakness	Debilidad
How would you describe the weakness?	¿Cómo describiría Ud. la debilidad?

When did you first notice the weakness?

¿Cuándo notó Ud. la debilidad por primera vez?

Did the weakness begin in the same muscles that feel weak now?

¿Comenzó la debilidad en los mismos músculos donde la tiene ahora?

Has the weakness increased?

¿Ha aumentado la debilidad?

Medical history

Have you ever injured your:

¿Se ha Ud. lastimado alguna vez un(a):

– bone?
– muscle?
– ligament?
– cartilage?
– joint?
– tendon?
  What was the injury?
  How did it happen?
  When did it happen?
  How was it treated?
  Do you have any problems as a result of the injury?

– hueso?
– músculo?
– ligamento?
– cartílago?
– articulación?
– tendón?
  ¿Cómo fue la lesión?
  ¿Cómo ocurrió?
  ¿Cuándo ocurrió?
  ¿Qué tratamiento se le dió?
  ¿Tiene algún problema a raíz de la lesión?

Have you had surgery or other treatment involving bones, muscles, joints, ligaments, tendons, or cartilage?
– What type of surgery or treatment did you have?
– What was the outcome?

¿Ha tenido Ud. cirugía u otro tratamiento del hueso, músculo, ligamento, tendón, cartílago o de la articulación?
– ¿Qué tipo de cirugía o tratamiento le realizaron?
– ¿Cuál fue el resultado?

Have you had X-rays of your bones?
– What bones were X-rayed?

– When did you have these X-rays?
– What did these X-rays show?

¿Se le han tomado radiografías de los huesos?
– ¿De qué huesos se tomaron las radiografías?
– ¿Cuándo se tomaron las radiografías?
– ¿Qué mostraron las radiografías?

Have you had blood or urine tests because of a muscle or bone problem?
– When?
– What were the results of these tests?

¿Se le han hecho análisis de sangre o de orina a causa de un problema muscular u óseo?
– ¿Cuándo?
– ¿Cuáles fueron los resultados de estos análisis?

Have you had fluid removed from a joint or had a biopsy?

¿Se le ha extraído líquido de las articulaciones (coyunturas) o se le ha hecho una biopsia?

– When?
– What were the results?

– ¿Cuándo?
– ¿Cuáles fueron los resultados?

What immunizations have you had?
– When did you have them?

¿Qué vacunas se ha dado?

– ¿Cuándo se las dió?

Do you have any other illnesses, such as:
– heart disease
– diabetes mellitus
– recent infections
– osteoporosis
– arthritis?

¿Tiene alguna otra enfermedad como:
– enfermedad cardiaca?
– diabetes mellitus?
– infecciones recientes?
– osteoporosis?
– artritis?

Family history

Has anyone in your family had:

¿Hay algún miembro de su familia que haya tenido alguna de las siguientes afecciones?

– osteoporosis?
– gout?
– arthritis?
– tuberculosis?
    Who?
    When?
    How was it treated?

– ¿osteoporosis?
– ¿gota?
– ¿artritis?
– ¿tuberculosis?
    ¿Quién?
    ¿Cuándo?
    ¿Qué tratamiento se le dió?

Health patterns

Medications

Medicamentos

Do you take any medications?
– Prescription?
– Over-the-counter?
– Home remedies?
– Herbal preparations?
– Other?

¿Toma Ud. medicamentos?
– ¿Con receta?
– ¿De venta libre?
– ¿Remedios caseros?
– ¿Preparados herbales?
– ¿Otro?

Which prescription medications do you take?
– How often do you take them?

¿Qué medicamentos de receta toma Ud.?
– ¿Con qué frecuencia los toma?

Which over-the-counter medications do you take?
– How often do you take them?

¿Qué medicamentos de venta libre toma?
– ¿Con qué frecuencia los toma Ud.?

Why do you take these medications?

¿Por qué toma Ud. estos medicamentos?

How much of each medication do you take?

¿Cuál es la dosis que Ud. toma de cada uno de estos medicamentos?

How does each drug make you feel?

¿Cómo le hace sentirse cada uno de estos medicamentos?

Are you allergic to any medications?
- Which medications?
- What happens when you have an allergic reaction?

¿Es Ud. alérgico(a) a determinados medicamentos?
- ¿Qué medicamentos?
- ¿Qué le pasa cuando tiene una reacción alérgica?

Personal habits

Hábitos personales

Do you smoke or chew tobacco?
- What do you smoke?
    Cigarettes?
    Cigars?
    Pipe?
- How long have you smoked or chewed tobacco?
- How many cigarettes, cigars, or pipes of tobacco do you smoke each day?
- How much tobacco do you chew each day?
- Did you ever stop?

    For how long?

    What made you want to stop?
    What method did you use to stop?
    Do you remember why you started again?

¿Fuma Ud. o masca tabaco?
- ¿Qué fuma Ud.?
    ¿Cigarrillos?
    ¿Cigarros (puros)?
    ¿Pipa?
- ¿Hace cuánto tiempo que Ud. fuma o masca tabaco?
- ¿Cuántos cigarrillos, cigarros (puros) o pipas de tabaco fuma Ud. al día?
- ¿Cuánto tabaco masca Ud. al día?
- ¿Dejó Ud. de fumar o mascar tabaco alguna vez?
    ¿Cuánto tiempo duró sin mascar o fumar tabaco?
    ¿Qué le hizo decidirse a dejar el hábito?
    ¿Qué método usó Ud. para dejar el hábito?
    ¿Recuerda Ud. por qué comenzó a usar tabaco otra vez?

If you do not use tobacco now, have you smoked or chewed tobacco in the past?

Si Ud. no consume tabaco actualmente, ¿ha fumado o mascado tabaco en el pasado?

Do you drink alcoholic beverages?
- What type?
    Beer?
    Wine?
    Hard liquor?
- How often do you drink alcoholic beverages?
- How many drinks do you have in one day?

¿Toma Ud. bebidas alcohólicas?

- ¿Qué tipo?
    ¿Cerveza?
    ¿Vino?
    ¿Aguardiente?
- ¿Con qué frecuencia toma bebidas alcohólicas?
- ¿Cuántos tragos toma en un día?

Spread over how much time?

¿Repartidas en cuánto tiempo?

Do you have any trouble urinating or moving your bowels?
- What type of problem are you having?

¿Tiene Ud. algún problema para orinar o defecar?
- ¿Qué tipo de problema?

Do you have trouble bathing or taking care of yourself?
- What kind of problems?
- How do you keep yourself clean and groomed?

¿Tiene problemas para bañarse o arreglarse?
- ¿Qué clase de problemas?
- ¿Cómo hace para mantenerse limpio y arreglado?

Do you have any problems writing?

¿Tiene problemas para escribir?

Sleep patterns

Patrones de sueño

Does your current problem make it hard for you to fall asleep?

¿El problema que Ud. tiene actualmente le trae problemas para dormirse?

Does the problem wake you during the night?
- How often does this happen?

¿Se despierta por la noche debido a su problema?
- ¿Con qué frecuencia ocurre esto?

Activities

Actividades

Do you have an exercise routine?
- What type of exercise do you do?
- How often do you exercise?

¿Sigue una rutina de ejercicios?

- ¿Qué tipo de ejercicio hace Ud.?

- ¿Con qué frecuencia hace Ud. ejercicio?

How has your current problem changed the way you exercise?

¿Cómo ha afectado su problema actual su manera de ejercitarse?

Have any of your usual activities, such as dressing, grooming, climbing stairs, or rising from a chair, become difficult or impossible?

¿Se han vuelto difíciles o imposibles algunas de sus actividades usuales, tal como vestirse, peinarse, subir escaleras o levantarse de una silla?

Do you use a cane, walker, or brace?

¿Usa un bastón, andador o aparato ortopédico?

Do you think using a cane, walker, or brace would help you walk?

¿Le parece que usar un bastón, andador o aparato ortopédico lo ayudaría a caminar?

Nutrition

How much coffee, tea, or other caffeine-containing beverages do you drink each day?

What do you usually eat in a 24-hour period?

How much do you weigh?
– Is this what you usually weigh?
– Have you recently gained or lost any weight?
  How much?

Does your current problem affect your ability to cook and eat?

Do you have trouble opening cans or cutting meat?

Sexual patterns

How does your current problem affect your sex life?

Environment

Do weather changes seem to make the problem better or worse?

Nutrición

¿Cuánto café, té u otras bebidas que contienen cafeína toma Ud. al día?

¿Cuál es su dieta típica en el transcurso de 24 horas?

¿Cuál es su peso actual?
– ¿Es éste su peso normal?
– ¿Ha aumentado o bajado de peso últimamente?
  ¿Cuánto?

Su problema actual, ¿afecta su capacidad de cocinar y comer?

¿Tiene Ud. dificultad para abrir latas o cortar carne?

Patrones sexuales

¿Qué efecto tiene este problema en sus relaciones sexuales?

Entorno

Los cambios climáticos, ¿parecen mejorar o empeorar el problema?

Psychosocial considerations

Coping skills

Does your current problem cause any stress?

How do you handle stress?

Roles

How do you feel about yourself?

Has this problem had a negative impact on your hobbies, activities, and social life?

– Please explain.

Habilidad de sobrellevar problemas

¿Se siente Ud. estresado por su problema actual?

¿Cómo manéja el estrés?

Roles

¿Cómo se siente consigo mismo(a)?

¿Ha tenido un efecto adverso este problema en sus pasatiempos favoritos, actividades y en su vida social?
– Explique.

What changes have you made because of this problem?	¿Qué ajustes ha tenido que hacer a raíz de este problema?

Responsibilities

Responsabilidades

What is your occupation?

¿Cuál es su profesión o trabajo?

Has your problem interfered with your ability to work?
– How?

¿Ha interferido su problema con su capacidad de trabajar?
– ¿Cómo?

Has your problem affected your responsibilities at home?
– How?

Su problema, ¿ha afectado sus responsabilidades en el hogar?
– ¿Cómo?

Developmental considerations

For the pediatric patient

Para el (la) paciente de pediatría

At what age did the child first:

¿A qué edad realizó la criatura los siguientes movimientos?

– hold up his or her head?
– sit?
– crawl?
– walk?

– ¿Sostener la cabeza levantada?
– ¿Sentarse?
– ¿Gatear?
– ¿Caminar?

Have you noticed that your child has problems with coordination?

¿Ha notado Ud. alguna falta de coordinación?

Can the child move normally?

¿Puede la criatura moverse de acá para allá normalmente?

Does the child seem to be as strong as other children his or her age?

¿Diría Ud. que la fuerza de la criatura es normal para su edad?

Has the child ever broken a bone?
– Which bone?
– When?
– How was it treated?
– Did any complications occur during the healing?

¿La criatura se ha quebrado alguna vez un hueso?
– ¿Cuál de ellos?
– ¿Cuándo?
– ¿Qué tratamiento recibió?
– ¿Se le desarrollaron complicaciones mientras sanaba?

For the pregnant patient

Para la paciente embarazada

Do you have pains or spasms in your back?
– How often do you have them?

¿Sufre dolores o espasmos en la espalda?
– ¿Con qué frecuencia los tiene Ud.?

- What do you do to relieve them?

Do you have a problem with:
- weakness?
- pain?
- tingling?
    How often does this problem occur?

- ¿Qué medidas toma Ud. para mitigarlos?

¿Tiene problemas al:
- debilidad?
- dolor?
- hormigueo?
    ¿Con qué frecuencia ocurre esto?

For the elderly patient

Para el (la) paciente anciano(a)

Have you broken any bones recently?
- Which bone?
- How did you break it?

¿Se ha quebrado algún hueso recientemente?
- ¿Qué hueso?
- ¿Cómo se lo quebró?

Have you noticed any change in your ability to move?

- What kind of change?

¿Ha notado Ud. algún cambio en su capacidad de movimiento?
- ¿Qué clase de cambio?

Do you exercise regularly?

- What type of exercise do you do?
- How often do you do it?

¿Hace Ud. ejercicio con regularidad?
- ¿Qué tipo de ejercicio hace Ud.?
- ¿Con qué frecuencia?

Have you gone through menopause?
- How old were you when you went through menopause?
- Are you taking estrogen?

¿Ha tenido Ud. la menopausia?
- ¿Qué edad tenía Ud. cuando tuvo la menopausia?
- ¿Toma Ud. estrógenos actualmente?

19

Immune system

Current health problems

Bleeding

Have you noticed any unusual bleeding?
– When did it start?

Where is the bleeding?
– Nose?
– Mouth?
– Gums?
– Cuts or lacerations?
– Other?

Have you noticed that you have bruises you do not remember getting?

Do you bruise easily?

Have you ever had a cut that bled for a long time?
– When did this happen?
– How did you stop the bleeding?

– How long did it bleed?

Have you vomited recently?

– What color was the material you vomited?
    Bright red?
    Coffee-colored?
    Black?
    Other?

Have you noticed any blood in your stools?
– What color were they?
    Bright red?
    Blood-streaked?

Sangrado

¿Ha notado Ud. algún sangrado anormal?
– ¿Cuándo le comenzó?

¿Dónde se encuentra?
– ¿En la nariz?
– ¿En la boca?
– ¿En las encías?
– ¿En cortes o laceraciones?
– ¿Otro?

¿Tiene moretones que no recuerda haberse hecho?

¿Le salen moretones con facilidad?

¿Ha sangrado Ud. por mucho tiempo a causa de un corte?
– ¿Cuándo ocurrió esto?
– ¿Cómo paró Ud. el flujo de sangre?
– ¿Cuánto tiempo sangró?

¿Ha vomitado Ud. últimamente?
– ¿De qué color era el vómito?

    ¿Rojo brillante?
    ¿Amarronado?
    ¿Negro?
    ¿Otro?

¿Ha notado Ud. sangre en su materia fecal?
– ¿De qué color era?
    ¿Rojo brillante?
    ¿Con vetas de sangre?

Black? | ¿Negro?
Other? | ¿Otro?

How often do you have blood in your stools?

¿Con cuánta frecuencia nota sangre en su materia fecal?

Have you noticed any change in the color of your urine?

¿Ha notado Ud. algún cambio en el color de la orina?

– What color was it? | – ¿De qué color era?
  Pink? | ¿Color rosado?
  Bright red? | ¿Rojo brillante?
  Other? | ¿Otro?
– Was the urine cloudy or clear? | – ¿Era la orina turbia o clara?
– How often does this color change happen? | – ¿Con cuánta frecuencia se produce este cambio de color?

Fatigue

Fatiga

Have you felt more tired than usual lately?

¿Últimamente se siente más cansado que lo habitual?

Are you tired all the time or only after a lot of activity?

¿Está Ud. cansado(a) todo el tiempo o sólo después de hacer mucha actividad?

Do you need to take naps?

¿Necesita dormir la siesta?

– How often do you nap? | – ¿Con qué frecuencia duerme Ud. la siesta?
– How long do you nap? | – ¿Por cuánto tiempo?

Fever

Fiebre

Have you had a fever recently?

¿Ha tenido Ud. fiebre últimamente?

– How high was your temperature? | – ¿A cuánto le subió la fiebre?

How often do you have a fever?

¿Con qué frecuencia tiene fiebre?

What do you do when you have a fever?

¿Qué hace cuando tiene fiebre?

Joint pain

Dolor de articulaciones

Do you ever have joint pain?

¿Tiene Ud. alguna vez dolor de articulaciones?

– In which joints? | – ¿Cuáles son las articulaciones (coyunturas) afectadas?
– How often does it occur? | – ¿Con qué frecuencia ocurre esto?

Describe the pain.

Describa el dolor.

– How long does it last? | – ¿Cuánto tiempo dura?
– What makes it better? | – ¿Qué mejora el problema?
– What makes it worse? | – ¿Qué lo empeora?

Do swelling, redness, or warmth occur with the pain?

¿Va el dolor acompañado de hinchazón, enrojecimiento o entibiamiento de la zona?

Sensory changes

Have you developed any vision problems recently?
- What kind of changes?
    Double vision?
    Increased sensitivity to light?

    Night blindness?
    Halos around lights?
    Vision loss?
    Other?
- When did you first notice these changes?

Has your hearing changed recently?
- How?
- When did you first notice the change?

Cambios sensoriales

¿Ha tenido Ud. problemas de visión últimamente?
- ¿Qué clase de cambios?
    ¿Visión doble?
    ¿Aumento de sensibilidad a la luz?
    ¿Ceguera nocturna?
    ¿Halos alrededor de luces?
    ¿Pérdida de visión?
    ¿Otro?
- ¿Cuándo los notó Ud. por primera vez?

¿Ha cambiado su audición últimamente?
- ¿Cómo?
- ¿Cuándo notó Ud. el cambio por primera vez?

Skin changes

Have you noticed any changes in your skin?
- What kind of changes?
    Texture?
    Color?
    Other changes?

Have you noticed any sores that heal slowly?
- Where were the sores?
- When did they develop?
- What did you do to help them heal?

Have you noticed any rashes or skin discoloration?
- Where?
- How long has your skin looked this wayt?

Cambios en la piel

¿Ha notado Ud. algunos de los siguientes cambios en su piel?
- ¿Qué tipo de cambios?
    ¿Textura?
    ¿Color?
    ¿Otro?

¿Ha notado llagas que sanan lentamente?
- ¿Dónde tiene Ud. las llagas?
- ¿Cuándo se le desarrollaron?
- ¿Qué medidas ha tomado Ud. para ayudarlas a sanar?

¿Ha notado Ud. alguna erupción o decoloración de la piel?
- ¿Dónde?
- ¿Hace cuánto tiempo que la tiene?

Swelling

Have you noticed any swelling in your:
- Neck?
- Armpits?
- Groin?

Hinchazón

¿Ha notado hinchazón en alguna de las siguientes áreas?
- ¿El cuello?
- ¿Las axilas?
- ¿La ingle?

When did you first notice the swelling?

¿Cuándo notó Ud. la hinchazón por primera vez?

Are the swollen areas sore, hard, or red?

¿Están las áreas hinchadas, adoloridas, duras o enrojecidas?

Is the swelling on one or both sides of your body?

¿Las tiene en un lado del cuerpo o en los dos?

Weakness

Debilidad

Do you ever feel weak?
– When?
– What makes it better?
– What makes it worse?

¿Se siente Ud. débil a veces?
– ¿Cuándo?
– ¿Qué lo hace sentir mejor?
– ¿Qué lo empeora?

Are you weak all the time or only at certain times?

¿Está Ud. débil todo el tiempo o sólo en determinados momentos?

Does weakness ever interfere with your ability to perform your usual daily tasks, such as cooking or driving a car?

¿Interfiere la debilidad con su habilidad de hacer sus quehaceres cotidianos, tal como cocinar o conducir el automóvil?

Medical history

How often do you see a doctor for a checkup?

¿Con qué frecuencia consulta a un médico para que le realice un control?

Have you had any trouble walking? Do you experience a pins-and-needles sensation?
– When did the problem start? What makes the problem better?
– What makes the problem worse?

¿Ha tenido problemas para caminar? ¿Experimenta una sensación de hormigueo?
– ¿Cuándo empezó esto?
– ¿Qué es lo que mejora el problema?
– ¿Qué es lo que empeora el problema?

Have you recently developed wheezing, runny nose, or difficulty breathing?

¿Ha tenido últimamente una respiración jadeante, goteo de la nariz o dificultad para respirar?

– When did it start?

– ¿Cuándo empezó?

Do you ever have rapid heartbeats?
– When?
– What makes the problem better?
– What makes the problem worse?

¿Tiene alguna vez las pulsaciones aceleradas?
– ¿Cuándo?
– ¿Qué es lo que mejora el problema?
– ¿Qué es lo que empeora el problema?

Do you have a persistent or recurrent cough or cold?
– Do you cough up sputum?
 How much?
 How often?
 What color is the sputum?

Does your chest hurt when you cough, breathe deeply, or laugh?
– Describe the pain.

Has your appetite changed recently?
– How has it changed?

Do you have nausea, gas, or diarrhea?
– How often?

Have you had sore throats frequently in the past?

Do you recall being seriously ill as a child or being sick for a long time and going to the doctor a lot?

Do you have any allergies?
– What causes them?
– Which symptoms bother you most?

Have you ever had asthma?

– When did it start?
– How is it treated?

Do you have an autoimmune disease, such as acquired immunodeficiency syndrome (AIDS)?
– Have you tested positive for human immunodeficiency virus (HIV)?
 When?
 Have you received treatment?

Have you had any other disorders or health problems?
– Describe them.

¿Tiene una tos o un resfriado constante?
– ¿Escupe Ud. esputo al toser?
 ¿Cuánto?
 ¿Con cuánta frecuencia?
 ¿De qué color es el esputo?

¿Siente Ud. dolor de pecho cuando tose, respira profundamente o se ríe?
– Describa el dolor.

¿Ha cambiado su apetito últimamente?
– ¿De qué manera?

¿Tiene Ud. náuseas, flatulencia o diarrea?
– ¿Con cuánta frecuencia?

¿Tuvo Ud. frecuentes dolores de garganta en el pasado?

¿Recuerda Ud. si de niño(a) estuvo enfermo(a) de gravedad o haber tenido una enfermedad prolongada e ir frecuentemente al médico?

¿Tiene Ud. alergias?
– ¿Qué es lo que las provoca?
– ¿Qué síntomas le molestan más?

¿Ha tenido Ud. asma alguna vez?
– ¿Cuándo comenzó?
– ¿Cómo fue tratado?

¿Sufre Ud. de alguna enfermedad autoinmune, tal como Síndrome de inmunodeficiencia adquirida (SIDA)?
– ¿Es Ud. seropositivo del Virus de inmunodeficiencia humano (VIH)?
 ¿Cuándo se hizo el análisis?
 ¿Ha recibido tratamiento?

¿Ha tenido Ud. otros trastornos o problemas de salud?
– Descríbalos.

Have you ever had surgery?

– What kind?
– When?
– What follow-up care did you receive?

Have you had an organ transplant?
– When?
– What kind of transplant did you have?
– What follow-up care did you receive?

Have you ever had a blood transfusion?
– When?
– Why?
– How many units of blood did you receive?
– Did you ever have a reaction?

Have you ever been rejected as a blood donor?
– Why?

Have you ever been in military service?
– When?
– Where did you serve?

¿Ha tenido Ud. cirugía alguna vez?
– ¿Qué tipo?
– ¿Cuándo?
– ¿Qué tratamiento complementario se le dió?

¿Se le ha transplantado algún órgano?
– ¿Cuándo?
– ¿Qué tipo de transplante le realizaron?
– ¿Qué tratamiento complementario se le dió?

¿Ha tenido Ud. alguna vez una transfusión de sangre?
– ¿Cuándo?
– ¿Por qué?
– ¿Cuántas unidades de sangre recibió?
– ¿Alguna vez tuvo una reacción?

¿Lo han rechazado alguna vez como donante de sangre?
– ¿Por qué?

¿Ha servido Ud. alguna vez en el ejército?
– ¿Cuándo?
– ¿Dónde hizo Ud. el servicio militar?

Family history

How would you describe the health of your blood relatives?

How old are your living relatives?

How old were those who died?

What caused their deaths?

Has anyone in your family had immune, blood, or other problems?

¿Cómo describiría Ud. la salud de sus parientes consanguíneos(as)?

¿Qué edad tienen sus parientes que aún viven?

¿A qué edad murieron los otros?

¿Qué fue lo que causó su muerte?

¿Tienen o tuvieron algunos de ellos problemas inmunológicos, de la sangre u otros?

Health patterns

Medications

Do you take any medication?
- Prescription?
- Over-the-counter?
- Home remedies?
- Herbal preparations?
- Other?

Which prescription medications do you take?
- How often do you take them?

Which over-the-counter medications do you take?
- How often do you take them?

Why do you take these medications?

How much of each medication do you take?

How does each medication make you feel?

Are you allergic to any medications?
- Which medications?
- What happens when you have an allergic reaction?

Have you ever used intravenous (I.V.) drugs?
- Which ones?
- When and why?

Personal habits

Do you smoke or chew tobacco?
- What do you smoke?
    Cigarettes?
    Cigars?
    Pipe?
- How long have you smoked or chewed tobacco?
- How many cigarettes, cigars, or pipes of tobacco do you smoke each day?

Medicamentos

¿Toma Ud. algún medicamento?
- ¿Con receta?
- ¿De venta libre?
- ¿Remedios caseros?
- ¿Preparados herbales?
- ¿Otro?

¿Qué medicamentos de receta toma Ud.?
- ¿Con qué frecuencia los toma Ud.?

¿Qué medicamentos de venta libre toma?
- ¿Con qué frecuencia los toma Ud.?

¿Por qué toma Ud. estos medicamentos?

¿Qué dosis toma Ud. de cada uno?

¿Cómo le hace sentirse cada uno de estos medicamentos?

¿Es Ud. alérgico(a) a determinados medicamentos?
- ¿Qué medicamentos?
- ¿Qué le pasa cuando tiene una reacción alérgica?

¿Ha usado Ud. drogas intravenosas?
- ¿Cuáles?
- ¿Cuándo y por qué?

Hábitos personales

¿Fuma Ud. o masca tabaco?

- ¿Qué fuma Ud.?
    ¿Cigarrillos?
    ¿Cigarros (puros)?
    ¿Pipa?
- ¿Hace cuánto tiempo que Ud. fuma o masca tabaco?
- ¿Cuántos cigarrillos, cigarros (puros) o pipas de tabaco fuma Ud. al día?

– How much tobacco do you chew each day?

– Did you ever stop?

    For how long?

    What made you decide to stop?

    What method did you use to stop?

    Do you remember why you started again?

If you do not use tobacco now, have you smoked or chewed tobacco in the past?

Do you drink alcoholic beverages?

– What type?

    Beer?

    Wine?

    Hard liquor?

– How often do you drink alcoholic beverages?

– How many drinks do you have in one day?

    Spread over how much time?

– ¿Cuánto tabaco masca Ud. al día?

– ¿Dejó Ud. de usar tabaco alguna vez?

    ¿Cuánto tiempo duró sin usarlo?

    ¿Qué lo hizo decidirse a dejar el hábito?

    ¿Qué método usó Ud. para dejar el hábito?

    ¿Recuerda Ud. por qué volvió a fumar o mascar tabaco otra vez?

¿Si Ud. no consume tabaco actualmente, ha fumado o mascado tabaco en en el pasado?

¿Toma Ud. bebidas alcohólicas?

– ¿Qué tipo de bebidas?

    ¿Cerveza?

    ¿Vino?

    ¿Aguardiente?

– ¿Con qué frecuencia toma bebidas alcohólicas?

– ¿Cuántos tragos toma en un día?

    ¿Repartidas en cuánto tiempo?

Sleep patterns

How many hours do you sleep each night?

When you wake up, do you feel rested?

Has your current problem affected your sleep pattern?

– How?

Patrones de sueño

¿Cuántas horas duerme por noche?

Cuando se despierta, ¿se siente bien descansado?

Su problema actual, ¿ha afectado su patrón de sueño?

– ¿Cómo?

Activities

Describe what you do every day.

Has your current problem affected your ability to do your usual activities?

– How?

Actividades

Describa lo que hace todos los días.

Su problema actual, ¿ha afectado su capacidad dde realizar sus actividades habituales?

– ¿Cómo?

Nutrition

What is your typical daily diet?

What kind of food and how much food do you eat at each meal?

What do you eat between meals?

Have you gained or lost weight recently?
– How much?
– Over what period of time?

Nutrición

¿Cuál es su dieta típica diaria?

¿Qué clase y qué cantidad de alimentos ingiere Ud. en cada comida?

¿Qué come Ud. entre las comidas?

¿Ha aumentado o perdido peso últimamente?
– ¿Cuánto?
– ¿En qué período de tiempo?

Sexual patterns

Are you sexually active?

– Do you have sex with more than one partner?

Do you use condoms?

Have you noticed any change in your sexual functioning?
– Can you describe this change?

Do you prefer having sex with:

– men?
– women?
– both?

Have you ever had anal sex?

Patrones sexuales

¿Tiene Ud. relaciones sexuales actualmente?
– ¿Tiene Ud. más de un(a) compañero(a)?

¿Utiliza condones?

¿Ha notado Ud. algún cambio en su desempeño sexual?
– ¿Puede Ud. describir este cambio?

Prefiere tener relaciones sexuales con:

– ¿hombres?
– ¿mujeres?
– ¿ambos?

¿Ha tenido sexo anal alguna vez?

Environment

Where do you work?

Are you exposed to any dangerous chemicals at work?
– What chemicals?
– How long have you been exposed to them?

Entorno

¿Dónde trabaja?

¿Está Ud. expuesto(a) a químicos peligrosos en el trabajo?
– ¿Cuáles son?
– ¿Hace cuánto que esta expuesto a esos químicos?

Psychosocial considerations

Coping skills

How would you rate your stress level?

What do you do to handle stress?

Have you recently had mood swings, been angry, or felt depressed?

Do your family members and friends give you emotional support?
– How do they perceive and cope with your illness?

Habilidad de sobrellevar problemas

¿Cómo clasificaría Ud. su nivel de estrés?

¿Qué hace para manejar el estrés?

¿Ha sufrido Ud. últimamente de inestabilidad emocional, irritabilidad o depresión?

Sus familiares y amigos, ¿le brindan apoyo emocional?
– ¿Cómo perciben y cómo se las arreglan con su enfermedad?

Responsibilities

What is your occupation?

Has your problem interfered with your ability to work?
– How?

Has your problem affected what you do at home?
– How?

Responsabilidades

¿Cuál es su profesión o trabajo?

¿Ha interferido su problema con su capacidad de trabajar?
– ¿Cómo?

Su problema, ¿ha afectado sus tareas en el hogar?
– ¿Cómo?

Developmental considerations

For the pediatric patient

Is the infant breast-fed or bottle-fed?

What type of formula do you use?

Does the child ever look pale or seem very tired?

Does the child sleep too much?

Has the child gained weight at a normal rate?

Para el (la) paciente de pediatría

¿El bebé es amamantado o se lo (la) alimenta con biberón?

¿Qué clase de fórmula usa Ud.?

¿Hay veces que la criatura se ve pálida o muy cansda?

¿Duerme la criatura demasiado?

¿Ha aumentado de peso la criatura en una proporción normal?

Did the mother have bleeding complications when the baby was born?

¿Tuvo la madre algunas complicaciones de sangrado cuando nació el bebé?

Were the parents' blood types Rh-compatible?

¿Era la sangre de los padres de tipo Rh-compatible?

Does the child have frequent or continuous severe infections?

¿Tiene la criatura infecciones graves con frecuencia o continuamente?

– What kinds of infections?
– How long do they last?
– How are the infections treated?

– ¿Qué clase de infecciones?
– ¿Cuánto tiempo le duran?
– ¿Qué tratamiento se da a las infecciones?

Does the child have any allergies?
– To what?

¿Tiene la criatura alguna alergia?
– ¿A qué?

Does anyone else in the family have allergies?
– To what?

¿Hay otro miembro de la familia que tenga alergias?
– ¿A qué?

Which immunizations has the child received?

¿Qué vacunas se han dado a la criatura?

For the adolescent patient

Para la paciente adolescente

Are you sexually active?

¿Tienes relaciones sexuales actualmente?

Do you use condoms to protect yourself from sexually transmitted diseases?

¿Usas condones para protegerte de enfermedades de transmisión sexual?

Have you had sexual contact with anyone who has acquired immunodeficiency syndrome (AIDS)?

¿Has tenido contacto sexual con alguien portador del sindrome de inmunodeficiencia (SIDA)?

Do you have anyone to talk to about sex?

¿Tienes alguien con quien hablar sobre sexo?

Have you ever bled from a cut for an extended period of time?

¿Alguna vez te sangró un corte por un período prolongado de tiempo?

For the pregnant patient

Para la paciente embarazada

Have you ever had sexual contact with anyone with acquired immunodeficiency syndrome (AIDS)?

¿Alguna vez tuvo contacto sexual con alguien portador del síndrome de inmunodeficiencia (SIDA)?

Have you been exposed to communicable diseases such as chickenpox?

¿Ha estado expuesta a enfermedades contagiosas como la varicela?

Did you receive immunizations as a child?
- Which ones?

Recibió vacunas de niña?

- ¿Quáles?

For the elderly patient

Para el (la) paciente anciano(a)

Do you take walks?
- How far do you walk?
- How often?

¿Sale a caminar?
- ¿Qué distancia camina?
- ¿Con qué frecuencia?

Do you have any difficulty using your hands?

¿Tiene Ud. alguna dificultad para usar las manos?

Do you ever have headaches, faintness, dizziness, ringing in the ears, or confusion?
- How often?

¿Alguna vez tiene Ud. dolor de cabeza, vahídos, mareos, zumbido en los oídos o confusión?
- ¿Con qué frecuencia le ocurren?

Have you ever had arthritis, osteomyelitis, or tuberculosis?
- When was it diagnosed?
- How was it treated?

¿Alguna vez ha tenido Ud. artritis, osteomielitis o tuberculosis?
- ¿Cuándo se le diagnosticó?
- ¿Qué tratamiento se le dió?

What do you eat on a typical day?

¿Qué come Ud. en un día típico?

Do you cook for yourself?

¿Cocina sólo para usted?

20

Endocrine system

Current health problems

Fatigue

How often do you feel tired?

– When did you first feel this way?
– Does anything make you feel better?

How would you describe this feeling?
– Constant?
– Intermittent?

Does this feeling seem to follow a pattern?
– What kind of pattern?

Mental status changes

Have you recently noticed any changes in your normal behavior, such as nervousness or mood swings?
– When did you first notice this?

How would you rate your ability to pay attention and remember things?

Muscle twitching

Have you noticed any muscle twitching?

– In which muscles?
– How often does this happen?

Fatiga

¿Con cuánta frecuencia se siente cansado(a)?
– ¿Cuándo se empezó a sentir así?
– ¿Hay algo que lo haga sentir mejor?

¿Cómo describiria esta sensación?
– ¿Constante?
– ¿Intermitente?

¿Parece esto seguir un patrón?

– ¿Qué tipo de patrón?

Cambios en el estado mental

¿Ha notado Ud. últimamente algún cambio en su conducta normal, tal como nerviosismo o cambios de humor?
– ¿Cuándo notó Ud. esto por primera vez?

¿Cómo calificaría su capacidad de prestar atención y recordar cosas?

Crispamiento espasmódico muscular

¿Ha notado Ud. algún crispamiento espasmódico muscular?
– ¿En qué músculos?
– ¿Con qué frecuencia se produce?

Endocrine system
El sistema endocrino

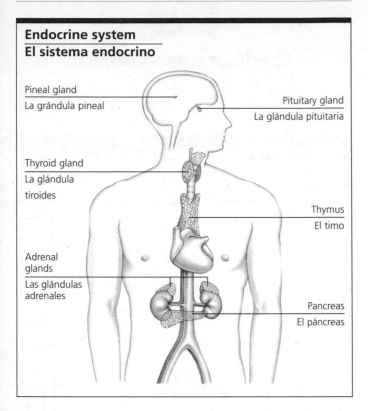

Pineal gland
La grándula pineal

Pituitary gland
La glándula pituitaria

Thyroid gland
La glándula
tiroides

Thymus
El timo

Adrenal
glands
Las glándulas
adrenales

Pancreas
El páncreas

– When did you first notice the twitching?	– ¿Cuándo notó Ud. el crispamiento por primera vez?
– How long does the twitching last?	– ¿Cuánto tiempo le dura el crispamiento?

Is it constant or intermittent?

¿Es constante o intermitente?

Does it seem to follow a pattern?

¿Parece seguir un patrón?

– What kind of pattern?

– ¿Qué tipo de patrón?

Do you have any numbness or tingling in your arms or legs?

¿Siente Ud. algún adormecimiento u hormigueo en los brazos o las piernas?

– How often?

– ¿Con cuánta fecuencia?

Polydipsia

Polidipsia

How much liquid do you drink each day?

¿Cuánto líquido bebe Ud. al día?

Have you been unusually thirsty lately?

¿Ha tenido más sed que la habitual últimamente?

– When did you first notice this?

– ¿Cuándo notó Ud. esto por primera vez?

Polyuria

How many times do you urinate each day?

Have you noticed an increase in the amount of urine you pass?
– How much of an increase?
– When did you first notice this?

Poliuria

¿Cuántas veces al día orina Ud.?

¿Ha notado un aumento en la cantidad de orina que Ud. expulsa?
– ¿Cuánto ha aumentado?
– ¿Cuándo notó Ud. esto por primera vez?

Weakness

Do you feel weak?
– When did you first feel weak?

– What makes it better?
– What makes it worse?

Is it constant or intermittent?

Do you feel weak all over or in a specific part of your body?

– Which part?

Debilidad

¿Se siente Ud. débil?
– ¿Cuándo notó Ud. esto por primera vez?
– ¿Qué mejora el problema?
– ¿Qué lo empeora?

¿Es constante o intermitente?

¿Es la debilidad general o se limita a una zona específica del cuerpo
– ¿A qué zona?

Medical history

Have you ever fractured your skull or repeatedly broken other bones?
– When did this happen?
– How was it treated?

Have you ever had surgery?

– When?
– Why?
– Did you have any complications after the surgery?

Have you ever had radiation treatments?
– When?
– Why?

Have you ever had a brain infection, such as meningitis or encephalitis?
– When?
– How was it treated?

¿Se ha fracturado Ud. el cráneo alguna vez o ha tenido repetidas fracturas en otros huesos?
– ¿Cuándo?
– ¿Qué tratamiento recibió?

¿Ha tenido Ud. cirugía alguna vez?
– ¿Cuándo?
– ¿Por qué?
– ¿Sufrió Ud. complicaciones después de la cirugía?

¿Ha recibido Ud. alguna vez tratamientos de radiación?
– ¿Cuándo?
– ¿Por qué?

¿Ha tenido Ud. alguna vez una infección del cerebro, tal como meningitis o encefalitis?
– ¿Cuándo?
– ¿Qué tratamiento se le dió?

Were you ever considered tall or short for your age?
- Did you have any growth spurts?
  When?
  How much did you grow?

¿Alguna vez se lo(a) consideró alto(a) o bajo(a) para su edad?
- ¿Hubo momentos en que Ud. creció de repente?
  ¿Cuándo?
  ¿Cuánto creció?

Have you ever been told you have an endocrine or glandular problem?
- What was the problem?
- When was it diagnosed?
- How was it treated?

¿Se le ha dicho alguna vez que tiene un problema endocrino o glandular?
- ¿Cuál fue el problema?
- ¿Cuándo se le diagnosticó?
- ¿Qué tratamiento se le dió?

Have you had any skin changes, such as acne, increased or decreased oiliness or dryness, or changes in color?
- When?

¿Ha tenido cambios de la piel, tal como acné, aumento o disminución de la oleosidad o sequedad o cambio de color?
- ¿Cuándo?

Do you bruise more easily than you used to?

¿Le salen moretones con mayor facilidad que antes?

Have you noticed any increase in the size of your hands or feet?

¿Ha notado Ud. algún aumento en el tamaño de las manos o de los pies?

Do your fingernails and toenails break easily?
- Have they thickened or separated from your fingers and toes?

¿Sus uñas de las manos y de los pies están quebradizas?
- ¿Ha aumentado el grosor de las uñas o se han separado de los dedos de la mano y del pie?

Have you noticed any change in how much body hair you have and where you have it?
- What kind of change?
- When did you notice the change?

¿Ha notado Ud. algún cambio en la cantidad de vello corporal y su distribución en el cuerpo?
- ¿Qué tipo de cambio?
- ¿Cuándo notó el cambio?

Has your voice deepened or changed in some other way?

- How?

Su voz, ¿es más grave que antes o ha cambiado de alguna otra manera?
- ¿Cómo?

Have you ever had neck pain?

- Describe it.

¿Ha tenido Ud. alguna vez dolor de cuello?
- ¿Descríbalo.

Has the size of your neck changed?
- In what way?
- When did you notice this change?

¿Ha cambiado el tamaño de su cuello?
- ¿De qué manera?
- ¿Cuándo notó este cambio?

Have you had any visual problems, such as double or blurred vision?
– Describe the problem.

¿Ha tenido Ud. algunos problemas de visión, tal como visión doble o nublada?
– ¿Describa el problema.

Do your eyes ever burn or feel "gritty" when you close them?

– When does this happen?

¿Hay veces en que los ojos le arden o se sienten "arenosos" cuando Ud. los cierra?
– ¿Cuándo ocurre esto?

Have you ever felt as though your heart was racing for no reason?
– How often?
– How long did it last?

¿Alguna vez sintió que el corazón le latía a un ritmo exagerado sin motivo?
– ¿Con cuánta frecuencia?
– ¿Cuánto duró la sensación?

Have you ever been told you have high blood pressure?
– When?
– How was it treated?

¿Se le ha dicho alguna vez que tiene presión sanguínea alta?
– ¿Cuándo?
– ¿Qué tratamiento se le dió?

Have you ever had seizures?

– What type?
– What was happening when you had your seizures?

¿Ha tenido Ud. convulsiones alguna vez?
– ¿De qué tipo?
– ¿En qué circunstancias se produjeron las convulsiones?

Do you often have headaches?

– How often?
– Describe them.
– How are they treated?

¿Tiene Ud. dolores de cabeza con frecuencia?
– ¿Con qué frecuencia?
– Descríbalos.
– ¿Cómo se los trata?

Family history

Does anyone in your family have:

– Diabetes mellitus?
– Thyroid disease?

– High blood pressure?
– Elevated blood fats?

   Who?
   When was it diagnosed?
   How was it treated?

¿Hay algún miembro de su familia que sufra de alguna de las siguientes afecciones?
– ¿Diabetes melitus?
– ¿Enfermedad de la glándula tiroides?
– ¿Alta presión sanguínea?
– ¿Sangre con alto nivel de adiposidad?
      ¿Quién?
      ¿Cuándo se le diagnosticó?
      ¿Qué tratamiento se le dió?

Health patterns

Medications

Do you take any medications?
– Prescription?
– Over-the-counter?
– Home remedies?
– Herbal preparations?
– Other?

Which prescription medications do you take?
– How often do you take them?

Which over-the-counter medications do you take?
– How often do you take them?

Why do you take these medications?

How much of each medication do you take?

How does each medication make you feel?

Are you allergic to any medications?
– Which medications?
– What happens when you have an allergic reaction?

Personal habits

Do you smoke or chew tobacco?
– What do you smoke?
   Cigarettes?
   Cigars?
   Pipe?
– How long have you smoked or chewed tobacco?
– How many cigarettes, cigars, or pipes of tobacco do you smoke each day?
– How much tobacco do you chew each day?
– Did you ever stop?

   For how long?

Medicamentos

¿Toma Ud. algún medicamento?
– ¿Con receta?
– ¿De venta libre?
– ¿Remedios caseros?
– ¿Preparados herbales?
– ¿Otro?

¿Qué medicamentos de receta toma Ud.?
– ¿Con qué frecuencia los toma?

¿Qué medicamentos de venta libre toma?
– ¿Con qué frecuencia los toma?

¿Por qué toma Ud. estos medicamentos?

¿Cuál es la dosis para cada uno de ellos?

¿Cómo le hace sentirse cada uno de estos medicamentos?

¿Es Ud. alérgico(a) a algunos medicamentos?
– ¿A qué medicamentos?
– ¿Qué le pasa cuando tiene una reacción alérgica?

Hábitos personales

¿Fuma Ud. o masca tabaco?

– ¿Qué fuma Ud.?
   ¿Cigarrillos?
   ¿Cigarros (puros)?
   ¿Pipa?
– ¿Hace cuánto tiempo que fuma o masca tabaco?
– ¿Cuántos cigarrillos, cigarros (puros) o pipas de tabaco fuma Ud. al día?
– ¿Cuánto tabaco masca Ud. al día?
– ¿Dejó Ud. de fumar o mascar tabaco alguna vez?
   ¿Cuánto tiempo duró sin fumar o mascar tabaco?

What made you decide to stop?

What method did you use to stop?

Do you remember why you started again?

¿Qué lo hizo decidirse dejar el hábito?

¿Qué método usó Ud. para dejar el hábito?

¿Recuerda Ud. por qué volvió a fumar o mascar tabaco?

If you do not use tobacco now, have you smoked or chewed tobacco in the past?

¿Si Ud. no consume tabaco actualmente, ha fumado o mascado tabaco en el pasado?

Do you drink alcoholic beverages?
– What type?
    Beer?
    Wine?
    Hard liquor?
– How often do you drink alcoholic beverages?
– How many drinks do you have in one day?
    Spread over how much time?

¿Toma Ud. bebidas alcohólicas?
– ¿Qué clase de bebidas?
    ¿Cerveza?
    ¿Vino?
    ¿Aguardiente?
– ¿Con qué frecuencia toma bebidas alcohólicas?
– ¿Cuántos tragos toma en un día?
    ¿Repartidas en cuánto tiempo?

Sleep patterns

Have you been sleeping more or less than usual?

Do you wake up at night to urinate?
– How often does this happen?

Hábitos de dormir

¿Está durmiendo más o menos de lo usual?

¿Se despierta Ud. por la noche para orinar?
– ¿Con qué frecuencia ocurre esto?

Activities

Do you exercise?
– How often?

What type of exercise do you do?

Have you had any difficulty exercising lately?

Actividades

¿Hace Ud. ejercicio?
– ¿Con cuánta fecuencia?

¿Qué tipo de ejercicio hace Ud.?

¿Ha tenido Ud. dificultad en hacer ejercicio últimamente?

Nutrition

Has your appetite increased or decreased recently?
– When did you first notice the change?

Nutrición

¿Ha aumentado o disminuido su apetito últimamente?
– ¿Cuándo notó Ud. el cambio por primera vez?

What did you normally eat in a day before your appetite changed?

¿Qué comía Ud. en el curso de un día antes que cambiara su apetito?

What do you eat now?

¿Qué come Ud. en la actualidad?

Have you recently gained weight without trying?

¡Ha aumentado Ud. de peso últimamente sin haber tenido la intención?

– How much?
– Over what time period?

– ¿Cuánto?
– ¿Durante cuánto tiempo?

Have you recently lost weight without trying?

¡Ha bajado Ud. de peso últimamente sin haber tenido la intención?

– How much?
– Over what time period?

– ¿Cuánto?
– ¿Durante cuánto tiempo?

Sexual patterns

Patrones sexuales

Has your current problem affected your sex life?
– How?

Su problema actual, ¿ha afectado su vida sexual?
– ¿Cómo?

Environment

Extorno

Have you been exposed to any chemicals or toxins?
– Which chemicals or toxins?
– For how long were you exposed?

¡Ha estado expuesto(a) a químicos o toxinas?
– ¿Qué químicos o toxinas?
– ¿Por cuánto tiempo estuvo expuesto(a)?

Psychosocial considerations

Coping skills

Habilidad de sobrellevar problemas

Are you less interested in people, things, and activities than you used to be?

¿Tiene Ud. menos interés que antes en las personas, las cosas y las actividades?

Do you ever feel depressed for no particular reason?

¿Se siente Ud. a veces deprimido(a) sin tener algún motivo?

Do you feel like you are under more stress than usual?

¿Siente que está bajo mayor estrés que el habitual?

Can you talk about what might be causing this stress?

¿Puede Ud. hablar sobre lo que podría estar provocándole este estrés?

Could stress be causing your current health problem?

¿Cree que el estrés sea la causa de su problema de salud actual?

Roles

What do you think of yourself?

Do you think your health problem will get better or worse?

What bothers you most about this problem?

Can you ask family members or close friends for help when you need it?

Roles

¿Qué opinión tiene sobre sí mismo(a)?

¿Cree Ud. que su problema de salud mejorará o empeorará?

¿Qué es lo que más le molesta de su problema?

¿Tiene Ud. miembros de la familia o amigos(as) íntimos(as) a quienes pedirles ayuda si la necesita?

Responsibilities

What is your occupation?

Does your current health problem interfere with your work?

Does your current health problem interfere with your responsibilities at home?

Responsabilidades

¿Cuál es su profesión o su trabajo?

¿Interfiere con su trabajo su problema actual?

Su problema de salud actual, ¿interfiere con sus responsabilidades en el hogar?

Developmental considerations

For the pediatric patient

Has the child's activity level changed?
– Describe a typical day before this change and a typical day now.

Have you ever been told that the child's growth and development are above or below normal rates?
– Who told you?

Has the child lost weight, been extremely thirsty or hungry, or been urinating frequently?

– When did you first notice these changes?

Para el (la) paciente de pediatría

¿Ha cambiado el nivel de actividad del (de la) niño(a)?
– Describa Ud. un día típico antes del cambio y un día típico en la actualidad.

¿Se le ha dicho alguna vez que el crecimiento y el desarrollo de la criatura es mayor o menor del promedio normal?
– ¿Quién se lo dijo?

¿Ha bajado de peso la criatura, ha tenido excesiva sed o hambre o ha orinado con frecuencia?

– ¿Cuándo notó Ud. estos cambios por primera vez?

For the pregnant patient

Have you ever been told you had diabetes during this or any other pregnancy?

Have you ever given birth to an infant weighing more than 10 pounds (4.5 kilograms)?
- How much did the infant weigh?

Para la paciente embarazada

¿Se le ha dicho que tiene diabetes durante este embarazo u otro embarazo previo?

¿Alguna vez dió a luz Ud. a un(a) infante(a) que pesó más de 10 libras (4.5 kilos)?
- ¿Cuánto pesó el (la) infante(a)?

For the elderly patient

Have you been extremely thirsty or hungry lately?

Have you been urinating more frequently than usual?

Are you taking any medication that may cause these sympptoms, such as a diuretic?

Para el (la) paciente anciano(a)

¿Ha tenido sed o hambre extremos últimamente?

¿Ha orinado con mayor frecuencia que la habitual?

¿Toma algún medicamento que puede provocar estos síntomas, como un diurético?

Appendices

Therapeutic drug classifications

Analgesic	Analgésico
Anesthetic	Anestésico
Antacid	Antiácido
Antiamebic	Agente antiamebiano
Antianginal	Agente contra anginas
Antiarrhythmic	Antiarrítmico
Antibiotic	Antibiótico
Anticancer agent	Agente anticarcinógeno
Anticoagulant	Anticoagulante
Anticonvulsant	Anticonvulsivo
Antidepressant	Antidepresivo
Antidiarrheal	Antidiarréico
Antiemetic	Antiemético
Antifungal	Antifúngico
Antigout agent	Agente contra la gota
Anthelmintic	Antihelmíntico
Antihemorrhagic	Antihemorrágico
Antihistamine	Antihistamínico
Antihypertensive	Antihipertensivo
Anti-inflammatory	Anti-inflamatorio
Antimalarial	Antimalaria
Antiparkinsonian	Antiparkinsoniano
Antipsychotic agent	Agente antipsicótico
Antipyretic	Antipirético
Antiseptic	Antiséptico
Antispasmodic	Antiespasmódico
Antithyroid agent	Agente antitiroides

Antituberculotic	Antituberculosis
Antitussive	Antitusígeno
Antiviral	Antiviral
Anxiolytic	Ansiolitico
Appetite stimulant	Estimulante para el apetito
Appetite suppressant	Supresor de apetito
Bronchodilator	Broncodilatador
Cardiac glycoside	Glucósido cardiaco
Decongestant	Descongestivo
Digestant	Digestivo (agente que estimula la digestión)
Disinfectant	Desinfectante
Diuretic	Diurético
Emetic	Vomitivo
Fertility agent	Agente para la fertilidad
Hematinic	Agente para aumentar la hemoglobina
Hypnotic	Hipnótico
Insulin	Insulina
Laxative	Laxante
Muscle relaxant	Relajante muscular
Oral contraceptive	Anticonceptivo oral
Oral hypoglycemic	Agente hipoglucémico oral
Oxytocic	Oxitócico
Sedative	Sedante
Steroid	Esteroide
Thyroid hormone	Hormona de la glándula tiroides
Tranquilizer	Tranquilizante
Vaccine	Vacuna
Vasodilator	Vasodilatador
Vitamin	Vitamina

Postoperative tubes, catheters, and equipment

After the surgery, you may have:

– more than one intravenous (I.V.) catheter in your arm.

– a catheter in your wrist, called an arterial line, to check your blood pressure and to measure oxygen levels in your blood.

– a tube in your bladder to drain your urine.

– a tube in your nose to drain fluids and acids from your stomach.

– an I.V. in the side of your neck or in your upper chest near your shoulder, called a central line.

– a tube in the side or middle of your chest to reinflate your lung or to drain fluid.

– a drainage tube inserted near the area where surgery was done to drain secretions.

– a very thin catheter in your back near your spine to give you pain medication.

– a device, with a little light taped or clipped to your finger or toe to measure oxygen levels.

– a dressing or bandage over your incision.

– stitches or metal clips, but no dressing or bandage over your incision.

– a blood pressure cuff wrapped around your upper arm and attached to a machine. It will

Después de la cirugía, Ud. puede tener:

– más de un catéter intravenoso (I.V.) en el brazo.

– un I.V. en la muñeca, que se llama línea arterial, para medir la presion sanguínea y el nivel de oxígeno en la sangre.

– un tubo en la vejiga para el drenaje de su orina.

– un tubo en la nariz para drenar fluidos y ácidos del estómago.

– un I.V. a un lado del cuello o de la parte superior del tórax cerca del hombro, que se llama línea central.

– un tubo a un lado o en medio del tórax para inflar el pulmón o para drenar fluido.

– un tubo de drenaje insertado cerca de la región donde se hizo la cirugía para el drenaje de secreción.

– un catéter muy fino en la espalda cerca de la columna vertebral para administrarle calmantes.

– un aparato, que se llama pulsoxímetro, con una pequeña luz fijado con cinta adhesiva o broches a un dedo de la mano o del pie.

– apósitos o vendajes para cubrir la incisión.

– puntos de sutura o clips de metal, pero sin apósitos o vendajes sobre la incisión.

– un manguito del tensiómetro alrededor de la parte superior del brazo y fijado a un aparato.

automatically inflate and deflate to measure your blood pressure and pulse.
– a little machine to supply pain medication through your I.V.

You may press the PCA every _____ minutes to give yourself extra pain medicine.

Se inflará y desinflará para medir automáticamente su presión sanguínea y su pulso.
– un pequeño aparato que provee medicamento contra el dolor a través de su I.V.

Ud. puede presionar el PCA cada _____ minutos para administrarse una dósis extra de calmante.

Medication
teaching phrases

This medication will:
– raise your blood pressure.
– improve circulation to your
_____.

– lower your blood pressure.
– lower your blood sugar.

– make your heart rhythm more
even.
– raise your blood sugar.

– reduce blood clots or prevent
them from forming.
– remove fluid from your body.
– remove fluid from your feet,
ankles, or legs.
– remove fluid from your lungs
so that they work better.
– remove fluid from your pancreas so that it works better.

**This medication will help your
body:**
– kill the bacteria in your _____.

– slow your heart rate.
– soften your bowel movements.
– raise your heart rate.
– use insulin more efficiently.

This medication will help you:

– breathe more easily.
– fight infections.
– relax.
– sleep.
– think more clearly.

Este medicamento hará que:
– su presión sanguínea suba.
– la circulación por
_____ (la región
del cuerpo) mejore.

– su presión sanguínea baje.
– el nivel de azúcar en la sangre
baje.

– el ritmo cardiaco sea más uni-
forme.
– su nivel de azúcar en la sangre
suba.

– se reduzcan los coágulos de
sangre o se evite su formación.
– elimine fluido del cuerpo.
– elimine fluido de los pies, tobillos o piernas.
– elimine fluido de los pulmones
para que funcionen mejor.
– elimine fluido del páncreas para
que funcione mejor.

**Este medicamento ayudará a
su cuerpo a:**
– destruir la bacteria del (de la)
_____ (región infecta-
da).
– reducir sus pulsaciones.
– ablandar sus evacuaciones.
– acelerar sus pulsaciones.
– usar la insulina más eficazmente.

**Este medicamento lo ayudará
a:**
– respirar con mayor facilidad.
– luchar contra infecciones.
– relajarse.
– dormir.
– pensar con mayor claridad.

This medication will reduce:

– the amount of acid your stomach produces.
– anxiety.
– bladder spasms.
– the burning sensation in your stomach or chest.
– the burning sensation when you urinate.
– diarrhea.
– muscle cramps.
– nausea.
– pain in your _____.

This medication will help your body produce more (less):

– antibodies.
– clotting factors.
– insulin.
– platelets.
– red blood cells.
– white blood cells.

This medication or treatment will destroy:

– antibodies.
– bacteria.
– cancer cells.
– clotting factors.
– platelets.
– red blood cells.
– white blood cells.

Este medicamento le aliviará o disminuirá:

– la producción de ácido en el estómago.
– la angustia.
– los espasmos en la vejiga.
– la sensasión de ardor en el estómago o tórax.
– la sensación de ardor al orinar.

– la diarrea.
– los espasmos musculares.
– las náuseas.
– el dolor en la (el) _____.

Este medicamento ayudará a su cuerpo a producir más o menos:

– anticuerpos.
– factores o agentes coagulantes.
– insulina.
– plaquetas.
– glóbulos rojos.
– glóbulos blancos.

Este medicamento o tratamiento destruirá:

– anticuerpos.
– bacterias.
– células cancerosas.
– factores o agentes coagulantes.
– plaquetas.
– glóbulos rojos.
– glóbulos blancos.

Home care phrases

Home safety	Seguridad en el hogar
Make sure walkways are well lit and clear of clutter.	Cerciórese de que los pasillos estén bien alumbrados y libres de objetos desparramados.
Remove throw rugs.	Quite todos los tapetes sueltos.
Repair handrails that are not sturdy.	Repare los pasamanos que no estén bien asegurados.
Handrails should run from the top of the stairs to the bottom.	Debe haber pasamanos en toda la escalera.
Never smoke in bed.	Nunca fume en la cama.
Never leave your cigarette, cigar, or pipe burning while you are out of the room.	Nunca deje encendido su cigarrillo, cigarro (puro) o pipa cuando salga del cuarto.
Place your commode near your bed.	Ponga su silla retrete cerca de su cama.
Set the water heater to the low setting.	Ajuste el calentador de agua en un nivel bajo.
Place a nonskid mat in your shower or tub.	Ponga un tapete antideslizante en la tina o regadera.
Use liquid soap in the shower. This will help you avoid a fall while trying to pick up a dropped bar of soap.	Use jabón líquido en la regadera para evitar resbalarse al tratar de recoger el jabón que se haya caído.
Clear up spills right away.	Limpie cualquier líquido derramado inmediatamente.
Store items you use most frequently at waist level so you can reach them easily.	Guarde las cosas que usa con más frecuencia a la altura de su cintura para poder alcanzarlas con facilidad.
Install deadbolt locks on outside doors.	Instale cerrojos de seguridad en las puertas que dan a la calle.
Mark keys so they are easy to identify.	Marque las llaves para identificarlas con facilidad.

Tack down carpet edges.

Los bordes de los tapetes deben estar bien sujetos.

Remove anything that can cause fires, falls, or other injuries.

Deshágase de cualquier elemento que pueda provocar incendios, caídas u otras heridas.

Post a list of emergency numbers near each phone.

Tenga una lista de los números de emergencia cerca de cada teléfono.

Keep a phone by your bed and in living areas.

Tenga un teléfono al lado de su cama y en espacios vitales.

Make sure all exits are not blocked.

Asegúrese de que ninguna salida esté bloqueada.

Remove electrical cords from under carpets and furniture legs.

No tenga cables eléctricos debajo de los tapetes o las patas de los muebles.

Replace frayed or cracked electrical cords.

Reemplace los cables eléctricos que estén raídos o agrietados.

Install a smoke detector on each level of your home.

Instale un detector de humo en cada piso de su casa.

Test the batteries in your smoke detector at least once per year.

Compruebe las baterías de sus detectores de humo por lo menos una vez al año.

Move curtains, rugs, and furniture away away from heaters.

Quite las cortinas, los tapetes y los muebles que estén cerca de los calentadores.

Place space heaters in places where they will not tip over.

Coloque los calentadores donde no se puedan caer.

Label cleaning liquids clearly and store them away from heat and food.

Ponga Ud. etiquetas legibles en los envases de líquidos para limpiar y guárdelos lejos del calor y los comestibles.

Dispose of old newspapers.

Deshágase Ud. de periódicos viejos.

Poor lighting, cords on the floor, clutter, and throw rugs can cause falls.

Poca iluminación cables en el suelo, objetos desparramados y tapetes movibles pueden causar caídas.

Medications

Medicamentos

Wash your hands before touching medications.

Lávese las manos antes de tocar los medicamentos.

Check the medication's label for the name and instructions about how much to take and how often to take it.

En el envase del medicamento verifique el nombre y las instrucciones sobre la dósis y la frecuencia en que se debe tomar el medicamento.

Check the expiration date on all medications.

Verifique la fecha de vencimiento del medicamento.

Store medications according to pharmacy instructions.

Guarde los medicamentos según las instrucciones de la farmacia.

Under adequate lighting, read labels carefully before taking any medication.

Bajo una luz adecuada, lea Ud. la etiqueta del medicamento con mucho cuidado antes de tomarlo.

Do not crush medication without first asking the doctor or pharmacist.

No triture el medicamento sin antes preguntar al doctor o farmacéutico.

Contact your doctor if a new or unexpected symptom or another problem appears.

Póngase en contacto con su doctor si un síntoma nuevo o inesperado u otros problemas se presentan.

Do not stop taking medication unless your doctor tells you to.

No deje de tomar el medicamento, salvo que se lo ordene su doctor.

Throw away outdated medications.

Deseche los medicamentos vencidos.

Never take someone else's medications.

Nunca tome Ud. los medicamentos de otra persona.

Keep a record of your current medications.

Lleve un registro de sus medicamentos actuales.

Miscellaneous home care

Diversos cuidados en casa

Do you have an advance directive?

¿Tiene Ud. una "Directiva anticipada"?

An advance directive is a legal document that directs your future health care in case you cannot speak for yourself.

Una "Directiva anticipada" es un documento que Ud. prepara ahora para dirigir su cuidado médico si no pudiera hablar por usted misma(o) en el futuro.

A living will outlines what you would like to be done if you are near death or in a coma.

Un testamento en vida señala el tratamiento que Ud. quisiera recibir si estuviera en coma o próximo(a) a morir.

A durable power of attorney for health care identifies the person you would like to make health care decisions for you if you are not able to make them for yourself.

Un poder no caducable para el cuidado de la salud identifica a la persona que Ud. quisiera que tomara decisiones por usted respecto de su atención médica en caso de que Ud. se encontrara incapacitado(a) para hacerlo.

Medicare will be responsible for your bill.

El seguro médico del Estado (Medicare) será responsable de su factura (cuenta).

What is your primary health insurance?

¿Cúal es su seguro principal de salud?

Do you have a job?

¿Tiene trabajo?

I will visit you again on Monday (Tuesday, Wednesday, Thursday, Friday, Saturday, Sunday).

Volveré a visitarla(lo) el lunes (martes, miércoles, jueves, viernes, sábado, domingo).

May I use your phone to call your doctor?

¿Me permite Ud. usar su teléfono para llamar a su doctor?

The home health aide will help you bathe and dress.

El (la) auxiliar sanitario(a) le ayudará a bañarse y vestirse.

Discharge and follow-up care

Alta y tratamiento complementario

When you are stable, you will be discharged to:

Cuando esté estable, será dado(a) de alta y trasladado(a) a:

– your home.
– a skilled care facility.

– su casa.
– una instalación especializada en el cuidado de la salud.

– a rehabilitation facility.

– una instalación de rehabilitación.

In case of an emergency, dial 911.

En caso de emergencia, llame al 911.

Call your doctor's office to make an appointment.

Llame al consultorio de su doctor para hacer una cita.

These are written discharge instructions.

Éstas son instrucciones escritas al darle de alta.

You need to have your blood drawn on _____.

Es necesario sacarle sangre el: _____ (día, fecha).

Do you have any questions?

¿Tiene alguna pregunta?

Complementary and alternative therapies

Herbs and supplements	Hierbas y suplementos
Acidophilus	Acidophilus
Allspice	Pimienta de Jamaica
Aloe	Áloe
Aloe vera	Áloe vera
Anise	Anís
Bay leaf	Hoja (seca) de laurel
Bergamot	Bergamota
Black cohosh	Cohosh negro
Black pepper	Pimienta negra
Black tea	Té negro
Blue cohosh	Cohosh azul
Capsaicin	Capsaicina
Caraway seed	Carvi
Carob	Algarroba
Catnip	Nébeda
Cayenne	Pimienta del ají de Cayena
Chamomile	Manzanilla
Chaparral	Chaparral
Chili pepper	Chile mexicano
Chinese medicine	Medicina china
Chondroitin sulfate	Sulfato de condroitina
Cilantro	Cilantro
Cinnamon	Canela
Clary sage	Salvia sclarea
Cocoa	Cocao
Comfrey	Consuelda

Cranberry	Arándano
Damiana	Damiana
Dandelion	Diente de león
Echinacea	Equinácea
Elderberry	Baya del saúco
Ephedra	Belcho
Eucalyptus	Eucalipto
Evening primrose	Onagra
Fennel	Hinojo
Feverfew	Matricaria
Flaxseed	Semilla de lino
Folate	Folato
Folic acid	Ácido fólico
Foxglove	Digital (dedalera)
Garlic	Ajo
Ginger	Jengibre
Ginkgo	Ginkgo
Ginkgo biloba	Ginkgo biloba
Ginseng −Asian −Serbian	Ginseng −Ginseng asiático −Ginseng servio
Goldenrod	Vara de oro
Goldenseal	Sello de oro
Glucosamine	Glucosamina
Grape seed	Semilla de uva
Green tea	Té verde
Hawthorn	Espino
Hazelnut	Avellana
Herbal medicine	Medicina herbal
Hyssop	Hisopo
Iron	Hierro
Kava kava	Kava kava
Lady's mantle	Pie de león *or* manto de la virgen

Lavender	Lavanda
Lemon	Limón
Lemon balm	Bálsamo de limón (Melissa)
Lemongrass	Limonicillo *or* lemongrass
Licorice	Orozuz *or* regaliz
Linden	Tilo
Ma huang	Ma huang
Marjoram	Mejorana
Marshmallow	Malvavisco
Melissa	Melissa
Mint	Menta
Milk thistle	Cardo de María (arzolla)
Mullein	Verbasco
Niacin	Niacina
Orange	Naranja
Oregano	Orégano
Panax ginseng	Ginseng panax
Paprika	Paprika
Parsley	Perejil
Passionflower	Pasionaria
Pau d'arco	Pau d'arco
Pennyroyal	Poleo
Peppermint	Pastilla de menta
Phospohorus	Fósforo
Plant estrogens	Estrógenos vegetales
Red clover	Trébol rojo
Rose hip	Rosa mosqueta
Rosemary	Romero
Rue	Ruda
Safflower	Alazor
Sage	Salvia
St. John's wort	Hierba de San Juan
Sarsaparilla	Zarzaparrilla

Sassafras	Sasafrás
Saw palmetto	Palma enana americana
Soy	Soja
Supplemental vitamins and minerals	Vitaminas y minerales complementarios
Tea	Té
Tea tree	Árbol de té
Thyme	Tomillo
Valerian	Valeriana
Vitamin(s)	Vitamina(s)
Wormwood	Ajenjo
Yarrow	Milenrama

Therapies	**Terapias**
Acupressure	Acupresión
Acupuncture	Acupuntura
Alexander technique	Técnica Alexander
Applied kinesiology	Kinesiología aplicada
Aromatherapy	Aromaterapia
Art therapy	Terapia artística
Ayurvedic medicine	Medicina Ayurvédica
Biofeedback	Bioretroalimentación
Breathing	Técnicas respiratorias
Chelation therapy	Terapia de quelación
Chiropractic	Quiropraxis
Colonic irrigation	Irrigación colónica
Color zone therapy	Cromoterapia
Counseling	Terapia psicológica
Craniosacral therapy	Terapia sacro-craneal
Crystal therapy	Terapia con cristales
Dance therapy	Danzoterapia
Deep breathing	Técnicas de respiración profunda
Diet – Gerson	**Dieta** – Gerson

– Macrobiotic	– Macrobiótica
Distraction therapy	Terapia de distracción
Fasting	Ayuno
Feldenkrais method	Método de Feldenkrais
Homeopathy	Homeopatía
Humor	Humor
Hydrotherapy	Hidroterapia
Hyperbaric oxygen therapy	Terapia hiperbárica de oxígeno
Hypnotherapy	Hipnoterapia
Ice application	Aplicación de hielo
Imagery	Formación de imágenes
Laughter	Risa
Light therapy	Terapia de luz
Magnetic field therapy	Terapia del campo magnético
Massage therapy	Terapia de masajes
Meditation	Meditación
Megavitamin therapy	Terapia de complejos vitamínicos
Moxibustion	Moxibustión
Music therapy	Musicoterapia
Naturopathy	Naturopatía
Polarity therapy	Terapia de polaridad
Qigong	Qigong
Reflexology	Reflexología
Reiki	Reiki
Relaxation techniques	Técnicas de relajación
Rolfing	Rolfing
Self-heal	Autocuración
Shiatsu	Shiatsu
Spiritual practices	Prácticas espirituales
Tai chi	Tai chi
Therapeutic touch	Toque terapéutico
Ultraviolet light therapy	Terapia de luz ultravioleta
Yoga	Yoga

Picture dictionary

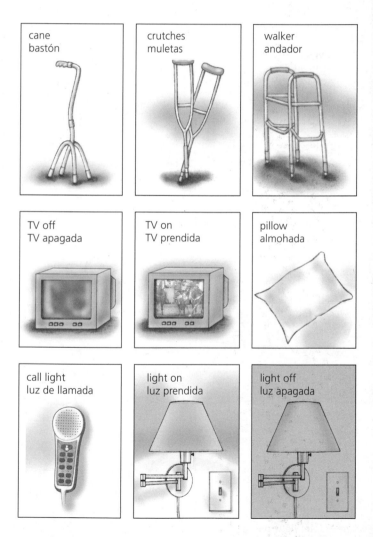

cane
bastón

crutches
muletas

walker
andador

TV off
TV apagada

TV on
TV prendida

pillow
almohada

call light
luz de llamada

light on
luz prendida

light off
luz apagada

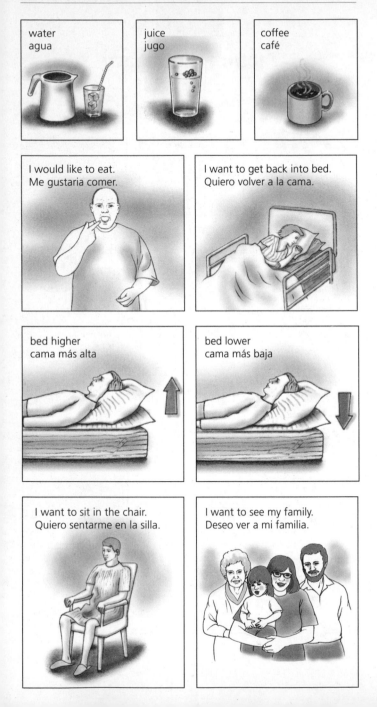

water
agua

juice
jugo

coffee
café

I would like to eat.
Me gustaria comer.

I want to get back into bed.
Quiero volver a la cama.

bed higher
cama más alta

bed lower
cama más baja

I want to sit in the chair.
Quiero sentarme en la silla.

I want to see my family.
Deseo ver a mi familia.

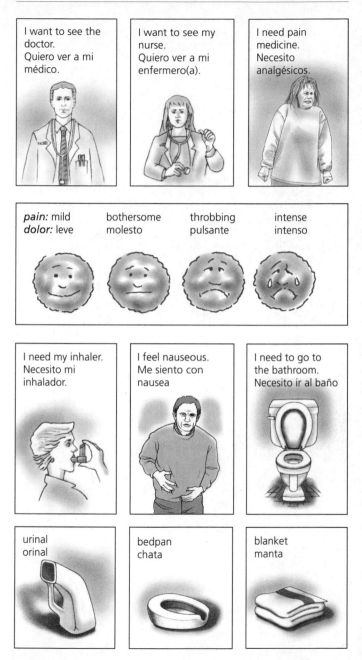

I want to see the doctor.
Quiero ver a mi médico.

I want to see my nurse.
Quiero ver a mi enfermero(a).

I need pain medicine.
Necesito analgésicos.

pain: mild
dolor: leve

bothersome
molesto

throbbing
pulsante

intense
intenso

I need my inhaler.
Necesito mi inhalador.

I feel nauseous.
Me siento con nausea

I need to go to the bathroom.
Necesito ir al baño

urinal
orinal

bedpan
chata

blanket
manta

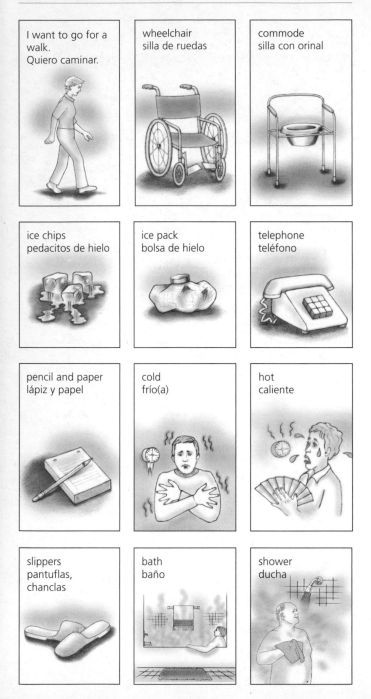

I want to go for a walk.
Quiero caminar.

wheelchair
silla de ruedas

commode
silla con orinal

ice chips
pedacitos de hielo

ice pack
bolsa de hielo

telephone
teléfono

pencil and paper
lápiz y papel

cold
frío(a)

hot
caliente

slippers
pantuflas, chanclas

bath
baño

shower
ducha

Pronunciation guide

English	Spanish	Pronunciation
abortion	el aborto	el aborto
abscess	el absceso	el abseso
addiction	la adicción	la adixeeon
adenoids	las adenoides	las adenoeedes
adenoma	el adenoma	el adenoma
anemia	la anemia	la anemeea
angina	la angina	la anheena
appendicitis	la apendicitis	la apendeeseetees
acquired immunodeficiency syndrome	el síndrome de inmunodeficiencia adquirida	el seendrome de inmoonode-feeseeeenseea adkeereeda
arteriosclerosis	la arteriosclerosis	la artereeosklerosees
arthritis	la artritis	la artreetees
asthma	el asma	el asma
backache	el dolor de espalda	el dolor de espalda
blindness	la ceguera	la segera
bronchitis	la bronquitis	la bronkeetees
burn (first-, second-, or third-degree)	la quemadura (de primer, segundo o tercer grado)	la kemadoora
bursitis	la bursitis	la boorseetees
cancer	el cáncer	el kanser
chest pain	el dolor de pecho	el dolor de pecho
chickenpox	la varicela	la vareesela
chills	los escalofríos	los eskalofreeos
cholesterol	el colesterol	el kolesterol

English	Spanish	Pronunciation
chorea	la corea	la korea
cold	el catarro, el resfriado	el katarro, el resfreeado
cold sores	las úlceras de la boca	las oolseras de la boka
constipation	el estreñimiento	el estreneemeeento
convulsion	la convulsión	la convoolseeon
cough	la tos	la tos
cramps	los calambres	los kalambres
deafness	la sordera	la sordera
diabetes	la diabetes	la deeabetes
diarrhea	la diarrea	la deearrea
diphtheria	la difteria	la deeftereea
discharge	el flujo	el floojo
dizziness	el vértigo, el mareo	el verteego, el mareo
eczema	el eccema	el exema
embolism	el embolismo	el emboleesmo
emphysema	el enfisema	el enfeesema
encephalitis	la encefalitis	la encefaleetees
epilepsy	la epilepsia	la epeelepseea
fainting spell	el desmayo	el desmajo
fatigue	la fatiga	la fateega
fever	la fiebre	la feeebre
fistula	la fístula	la feestoola
flu	la influenza, la gripe	la eenflooensa, la greepe
fluid	el fluido, el líquido	el flooeedo, el leekeedo
food poisoning	la intoxicación alimentaria	la eentoxeekaseeon aleementareea
fracture	la fractura	la fractoora
frostbite	la congelación	la kongelaseeon

English	Spanish	Pronunciation
gallbladder attack	el ataque de la vesícula biliar	el atake de la veseekoola beelear
gallstone	el cálculo biliar	el kalcoolo beelear
gangrene	la gangrena	la gangrena
gastric ulcer	la úlcera gástrica	la oolsera gastreeka
glaucoma	el glaucoma	el glaookoma
gonorrhea	la gonorrea	la gonorrea
hallucination	la alucinación	la alooseenaseeon
handicap	el impedimento	el eempedeemento
harelip	el labio leporino	el labeeo leporeeno
hay fever	la fiebre de heno	la feeebre de eno
headache	el dolor de cabeza	el dolor de kabesa
heart attack	el ataque al corazón	el atake al korason
heartbeat irregular rhythmical slow fast (tachycardia)	el latido irregular rítmico lento la taquicardia	el lateedo eerregoolar reetmeeko lento la takeekardeea
heartburn	las agruras (el ardor), la acedía	las agrooras (el ardor) la asedeea
heart disease	la enfermedad cardiaca	la enfermedad kardeeaka
heart failure	la insuficiencia cardiaca	la eensoofee-seeenseea kardeeaka
heart murmur	el soplo cardiaco	el soplo kardeeako
hemorrhage	la hemorragia	la emorrageea
hemorrhoids	las almorranas, las hemorroides	las almorranas, las emorroeedes
hepatitis	la hepatitis	la epateetees
hernia	la hernia	la erneea
herpes	el herpes	el erpes
high blood pressure	la presión alta	la preseeon alta
hit (on face)	el golpe (en el rostro)	el golpe en el rostro

English	Spanish	Pronunciation
hives	la urticaria	la oorteekareea
hoarseness	la ronquera	la ronkera
human immunodeficiency virus	el virus de inmunodeficiencia humano	el veeroos de eenmoonodefeesee-enseea oomano
ill	enfermo(a)	enfermo(a)
illness	la enfermedad	la enfermedad
immunization	la inmunización	la eenmoonee-saseeon
infantile paralysis	la parálisis infantil	la paraleesees een-fanteel
infarction	el infarto	el eenfarto
infection	la infección	la eenfexeeon
inflammation	la inflamación	la eenflamaseeon
injury	el daño, la lasti-madura, la herida	el daneeo, la las-teemadoora, la ereeda
itch	la picazón, la comezón	la peekason, la komeson
jaundice	la piel amarilla, la ictericia	la peeel amareesha, la eektereeseea
kidney stone	el cálculo en el riñón, la piedra en el riñón	el kalkoolo en el reeneeon, la peee-dra en el reeneeon
kidneys	riñones	reeneeones
laceration	la laceración	la laceraseeon
laryngitis	la laringitis	la lareengeetees
lesion	la lesión, el daño	la leseeon, el daneeo
leukemia	la leucemia	la leoosemeea
lice	los piojos	los peeojos
liver	el hígado	el eegado
lump	el bulto	el boolto
lungs	los pulmones	los poolmones
malaria	la malaria	la malareea

English	Spanish	Pronunciation
malignancy	el tumor	el toom_o_r
malignant	maligno(a)	mal_ee_gno(a)
malnutrition	la malnutrición	la malnootreesee_o_n
manic-depressive	maníaco-depresivo(a)	man_ee_ako depres-_ee_vo(a)
measles	el sarampión	el sarampee_o_n
medication	la medicina, el medicamento	la medees_ee_na, el medeekam_e_nto
meningitis	la meningitis	la meneeng_ee_tees
menopause	la menopausia	la menop_a_ooseea
menstruation	la menstruación	la menstrooasee_o_n
metastasis	la metástasis	la mat_a_stasees
migraine	la migraña, la jaqueca	la meegr_a_neea
mite	el ácaro	el _a_karo
mononucleosis	la mononucleosis infecciosa	la mononookle_o_sees eenfexee_o_sa
multiple sclerosis	la esclerosis múltiple	la eskler_o_sees m_oo_lteeple
mumps	las paperas	las pap_e_ras
muscular dystrophy	la distrofia muscular	la deestr_o_feea mooscool_a_r
mute	mudo(a)	m_oo_do(a)
myocardial infarction	el infarto cardiaco	el eenf_a_rto kard_ee_ako
myopia	la miopía	la meeop_ee_a
nephritis	la nefritis	la nefr_ee_tees
neuralgia	la neuralgia	la neoor_a_lgeea
obese	obeso(a)	ob_e_so(a)
obstruction	la obstrucción	la obstrooxee_o_n
ophthalmia	la oftalmia	la oft_a_lmeea
osteomyelitis	la osteomielitis	la osteomee-el_ee_tees
overdose	la sobredosis	la sobred_o_sees
overweight	el sobrepeso	el sobrep_e_so

English	Spanish	Pronunciation
pain	el dolor	el dolor
growing pain	el dolor de crecimiento	el dolor de creseemeeento
labor pain	el dolor de parto	el dolor de parto
phantom limb pain	el dolor de miembro fantasma	el dolor de meeembro fantasma
referred pain	el dolor referido	el dolor refereedo
sharp pain	el dolor agudo	el dolor agoodo
shooting pain	el dolor punzante	el dolor poonsante
burning pain	el dolor que arde	el dolor ke arde
intense pain	el dolor intenso	el dolor eentenso
severe pain	el dolor severo	el dolor severo
intermittent pain	el dolor intermitente	el dolor eentermeetente
throbbing pain	el dolor palpitante	el dolor palpeetante
painful	doloroso	doloroso
palpitation	la palpitación	la palpeetaseeon
palsy	la parálisis	la paraleesees
palsy, Bell's	la parálisis facial	la paraleesees faseeal
palsy, cerebral	la parálisis cerebral	la paraleesees serebral
paralysis	la parálisis	la paraleesees
Parkinson's disease	la enfermedad de Parkinson	la enfermedad de parkeenson
pellagra	la pelagra	la pelagra
pernicious anemia	la anemia perniciosa	la anemeea perneeseeosa
pertussis	la tos ferina	la tos fereena
pill	la píldora	la peeldora
pimple	el grano de la cara, el barrito	el grano de la kara, el barreeto
pneumonia	la pulmonía	la poolmoneea
poison ivy	la hiedra venenosa	la eeedra venenosa
poison oak	el roble venenoso	el roble venenoso
polio	la poliomielitis	la poleeomee-eleetees
polyp	el pólipo	el poleepo

English	Spanish	Pronunciation
postmenopausal	posmenopáusico(a)	posmeno-paooseeko(a)
premenopausal	premenopáusico(a) síndrome	premeno-paooseeko(a)
premenstrual syndrome	premenstrual	seendrome premenstrooal
psoriasis	la psoriasis	la soreeasees
pus	el pus	el poos
pyorrhea	la piorrea	la peeorrea
rabies	la rabia	la rabeea
rash	la roncha, el sarpullido, la erupción	la roncha, el sarpoosheedo, la eroopseeon
relapse	la recaída	la rekaeeda
renal	renal	renal
rheumatic fever	la fiebre reumática	la feeebre reoomateeka
roseola	la roséola	la roseola
rubella	la rubéola	la roobeola
rupture	la ruptura	la rooptoora
scab	la costra	la kostra
scabies	la sarna	la sarna
scar	la cicatriz	la seekatrees
scarlet fever	la escarlatina	la eskarlateena
scratch	el rasguño	el rasgooneeo
senile	senil	seneel
shock	el choque	el choke
sinus congestion	la congestión nasal	la kongesteeon nasal
sinuses	la sinusitis	la seenooseetees
slipped disk	el disco desplazado	el deesko desplasado
smallpox	la viruela	la veerooela

English	Spanish	Pronunciation
snakebite	la mordedura de culebra	la morded__oo__ra de kool__e__bra
sore	la llaga	la sh__a__ga
spasm	el espasmo	el esp__a__smo
spider bite	la picadura de araña	la peekad__oo__ra de __a__raneea
spotted fever	la fiebre maculosa	la fee__e__bre makool__o__sa
sprain	la torcedura	la torsed__oo__ra
stomach ache	el dolor del estómago	el dol__o__r de est__o__mago
stomach ulcer	la úlcera del estómago	la __oo__lsera del est__o__mago
suicide	el suicidio	el sooees__ee__deeo
sunburn	la quemadura del sol	la kemad__oo__ra de s__o__l
sunstroke	la insolación	la eensolasee__o__n
surgery	la cirugía	la seeroog__ee__a
swelling	la hinchazón	la eenchas__o__n
syphilis	la sífilis	la s__ee__feelees
tachycardia	la taquicardia	la takeek__a__rdeea
tapeworm	la lombriz solitaria	la lombr__ee__s soleet__a__reea
tetanus	el tétano	el t__e__tano
thrombosis	la trombosis	la tromb__o__sees
thrush	el afta	el __a__fta
tonsillitis	la tonsilitis, la amigdalitis	la tonseel__ee__tees, la ameegdal__ee__tees
toothache	el dolor de muela	el dol__o__r de moo__e__la
toxemia	la toxemia	la tox__e__meea
trauma	el trauma	el tr__a__ooma
tuberculosis	la tuberculosis	la tooberkool__o__sees
tumor	el tumor	el toom__o__r
typhoid fever	la fiebre tifoidea	la fee__e__bre teefoeed__e__a

English	Spanish	Pronunciation
typhus	el tifus, el tifo	el teefoos, el teefo
ulcer	la úlcera	la oolsera
unconsciousness	la pérdida del conocimiento	la perdeeda de konoseemeeento
undulant fever	la fiebre ondulante	la feeebre ondoolante
uremia	la uremia	la ooremeea
uterus, prolapsed	el prolapso de la matriz	el prolapso de la matrees
varicose veins	las venas varicosas, várices	las venas vareekosas, vareeses
venereal disease	la enfermedad venérea	la enfermedad venerea
canker sore	la postemilla	la postemeesha
chancre	el chancro	el chankro
chlamydia	la clamidia	la klameedeea
cold sore	los herpes labiales	los erpes labeeales
condyloma	el condiloma	el kondeeloma
cytomegalovirus	el citomegalovirus	el seetomegaloveeroos
genital herpes	el herpes genital	el erpes geneetal
genital wart	la verruga genital	la verrooga geneetal
gonorrhea	la gonorrea	la gonorrea
moniliasis	la moniliasis	la moneeleeasees
syphilis	la sífilis	la seefeelees
trichomonas	la tricomonas	la treekomonas
virus	el virus	el veeroos
vomit	el vómito, los vómitos	el vomeeto, los vomeetos
wart	la verruga	la verrooga
weakness	la debilidad	la debeeleedad
wheal	el verdugón, el moretón	el verdoogon, el moreton
wheeze	el jadeo, la sibilancia	el jadeo, la seebeelanseea
whiplash	la lesión de latigazo cervical	la leseeon de lateegaso serveekal
whooping cough	la tos ferina	la tos fereena

English	Spanish	Pronunciation
worm(s)	la lombriz (las lombrices)	la lombr<u>ee</u>s, las lombr<u>ee</u>ses
wound	la herida	la er<u>ee</u>da
yellow fever	la fiebre amarilla	la fee<u>e</u>bre amar<u>ee</u>sha

Cultural considerations for Hispanic patients

A patient's cultural beliefs can affect his attitudes toward illness and traditional medicine. By trying to accommodate these beliefs and practices in your care plan, you can increase the patient's willingness to learn and comply with treatment regimens. Because cultural beliefs may vary, individual practices may differ from those described here.

When caring for a Hispanic or Hispanic American patient, consider these common cultural beliefs and attitudes.

General health

– Patients may believe that health is influenced by environment, fate, and God's will.
– Patients may subscribe to Galen's theory, which states that the body's four humors—blood, phlegm, yellow bile, and black bile—must be kept in balance.
– Patients may believe in hot and cold theory of disease and health.
– Herbal teas and soup may be used as a patient recovers.
– A patient may express pain by nonverbal cues.
– Family may want to hide the seriousness of an illness from the patient.

Pregnancy and birth

– Pregnancy is considered a normal, healthy state.
– Pregnant patients may delay prenatal care and may prefer to use a *patera* or midwife.
– During labor and birth, women may be strongly influenced by the mother and mother-in-law and may not listen to the husband.
– Crying or shouting out during labor is acceptable behavior.
– After childbirth, the mother's legs are brought together to prevent air from entering uterus.
– The mother may wear a religious necklace that's placed around the neonate's neck after birth.
– New mothers may be restricted to boiled milk and toasted tortillas for the first 2 days after birth and may remain on bed rest for 3 days after birth.
– Postpartum patients may delay bathing for 14 days after childbirth.
– Postpartum patients may delay breast-feeding because colostrum is considered dirty and spoiled.
– Male neonates aren't circumcised.

Resources for Spanish-speaking patients

These agencies either have a focus on Hispanic health care issues or have information available in Spanish.

Administration on Aging
www.aoa.gov

Al-Anon Family Group Headquarters, Inc.
www.al-anon.org

American Cancer Society
www.cancer.org/docroot/esp/
esp_0.asp

American Diabetes Association
www.diabetes.org/espanol

American Lung Association
www.lungusa.org/espanol

American Red Cross
www.redcross.org
www.cruzrojaamericana.org

Aplastic Anemia & MDS International Foundation, Inc.
www.aamds.org

Centers for Disease Control and Prevention
www.cdc.gov/spanish/

Centers for Medicaid and Medicare Serives
www.medicare.gov/Spanish/
Overview.asp

Latina Share
www.sharecancersupport.org

Latino Organization for Liver Awareness (L.O.L.A.)
www.lola-national.org

March of Dimes Birth Defects Foundation
www.nacersano.org

MedlinePlus: Hispanic American Health
www.nlm.nih.gov/
medlineplus/
hispanicamericanhealth.html

National Alliance for Hispanic Health
www.hispanichealth.org

Office of Minority Health Resource Center
www.omhrc.gov

Project Inform
www.projinf.org/spanish/index.
html

Index

i refers to an illustration.

---

i refers to an illustration.

---

i refers to an illustration.

i refers to an illustration.

i refers to an illustration.

WXYZ

Walk, 248
Walker, 42, 203, 245
Walking patterns, 182, 185, 218
Weakness, muscular, 199-200,
     210, 221
Weight gain or loss, 54, 135, 160
Weight units, 14
Wheelchair, 248
Wheezing, 210
Whirlpool bath, 52
Work, types of, 8
Wound care, 30
  equipment for, 51-52
X-ray, 34, 37-38
  in cardiovascular system problems,
     122
  in musculoskeletal system
     problems, 200
  in respiratory problems, 108
Yoga, 244

Indice

i se refiere a una ilustración (lamina).

i se refiere a una ilustración (lamina).

i se refiere a una ilustración (lamina).

---

i se refiere a una ilustración (lamina).

i se refiere a una ilustración (lamina).

i se refiere a una ilustración (lamina).

i se refiere a una ilustración (lamina).
